Understanding China

The series will provide you with in-depth information on China's social, cultural and economic aspects. It covers a broad variety of topics, from economics and history to law, philosophy, cultural geography and regional politics, and offers a wealth of materials for researchers, doctoral students, and experienced practitioners.

Jie Wu

Politicized Medical Dispute Resolution in China

Springer

Jie Wu
Department of Political Science
Fudan University
Shanghai, China

ISSN 2196-3134 ISSN 2196-3142 (electronic)
Understanding China
ISBN 978-981-97-6960-5 ISBN 978-981-97-6961-2 (eBook)
https://doi.org/10.1007/978-981-97-6961-2

This Springer imprint is published by the registered company Springer Nature Singapore Pte Ltd.
The registered company address is: 152 Beach Road, #21-01/04 Gateway East, Singapore 189721, Singapore

To my parents
陆雁、吴国平
for their unconditional love

Acknowledgements

It might be a mistake to start my journey of Ph.D. I was unprepared for the endless self-doubts and rejections throughout my doctoral and future life, yet everyone I met made my life bliss. The four-year Ph.D. life familiarizes me with saying goodbye and settling down in a new place frequently. My calendar in Hong Kong "resets" every June, since many of my friends graduate and leave Hong Kong every summer. We accompany each other going through the ups and downs together during our time overlap and depart for our new destinations.

The final year in Cambridge makes my Ph.D. period more complete. I would like to thank my thesis writing buddies—Shiyu Zhang, Miaoyan Yang, Shen Yang, Yihui Su, and other Harvard-Yenching scholars. You all made my life abroad more like home. I realize the fact that smart people are always even more hard working. The key to surviving the academic life not only counts on the idea but implementation and diligence. I would memorize all day and night that we spent in Divinity 2, and the time at the Harvard-Yenching Library was also the best studying place for finishing the dissertation. Thanks, James Flaherty, Ruohong Li, Lindsay Strogatz, and Francesca Coppola for making my life here joyful and plentitude.

Many thanks to my supervisor, Dr. Helen Liu, for coaching me and proofreading my working paper to make it a better one. Special thanks to my "sister" group members Yiran Li, Kailin, and Nielin for better preparing me to be a Ph.D. Thanks, Dr. Zhu Jiangnan, Dr. Kwan Nok Chan, Dr. Quek Kai, Dr. Xiaoqi Wang, and Dr. Peter Cheung for your insightful comments and suggestions to my research. Thanks to my friends and teachers from Fudan University, which is the very beginning of my journey. Thanks, Dr. Arthur Kleinman, Dr. Tom Christensen, and Dr. Lawrence Reardon for providing detailed comments and enlightening suggestions to make my work more presentable and publishable.

Thank my friends for always being supportive. Tremendous thanks are also due to my friend Can Cui for pushing, supporting, and appraising me whenever I was down and sentimental. Thanks also go to Nai'er Tang for listening to my complaints, gossips when I am in Hong Kong, Shanghai, and Boston. It is always good to have a friend. Thanks, Huang Jie, Yexin Mao, Hanyu Chen, Xin Ge, and my cohort Al-Sudairi Mohammed Turki A., Mike Sadler, Han Xiao, Catherine Chen, Annie Song,

Lingbo Zhao, Siqin Kang, Daiding Zhang, Nikolai, Yudi, Felix, and Winston for making the office room 8.26 a better one. I would also like to thank my roommates and hallmates at Swire and GH: Li Qian, Zhang Yin, and Guo Yumeng for delighting my life in Hong Kong. I remember the past years we spent exploring the city and dining together. My first friend in Hong Kong Li Qian is the warmest and nicest person I know.

My research was also supported by the Swire Scholarship and Harvard-Yenching Institute. During my fieldwork, I also received a lot of help from scholars and government officials. I am indebted to Herb Zhang and the Springer team for their editorial help and keen insights. I would like to thank my teachers and colleagues at the Fudan University. You always set the role models for me to follow.

Last but not least, I am most indebted to my parents for supporting my decisions to change my life. I always refrain from showing my emotion every time at the airport for fear of making you even sad. I wish I could live up to your expectations. Your endless and unconditional love is the strongest support and shelter for me, wherever I am. Glad I am now back.

Contents

1 Introduction 1
1.1 Puzzle 3
1.2 Political Participation and Institutional Responses in China 6
1.3 Background: A Brief Historical Account of the Chinese Health System 13
1.4 Methods 18
1.5 Overview of the Book 20
References 22

2 Politicized Medical Dispute Resolution 29
2.1 Medical Dispute Resolution in the 1990s: Throw an Egg to the Stone 30
2.2 A Fragmented Medical Dispute Resolution Landscape in the Transition Era 33
2.3 Integrated Stability Maintenance Mechanism 38
2.3.1 Evolved Social Stability Mechanism 38
2.3.2 Institutional Change in People's Mediation Institutions in China 41
2.4 Institutional Constraints of Mediation Institutions and Politicalized Outcomes 45
2.4.1 Rule of Law 47
2.4.2 Social Power: Asymmetric Social Power Between Mediators and Disputants 49
2.4.3 Political Concern: Stability Maintenance 52
2.5 Summary 53
References 54

3 Understanding Hospital Violence in China 57
3.1 From "Empty Nose Syndrome" to Hospital Violence 57
3.2 Methods 60
3.3 Hospital Violence as a Form of Resistance 62

3.3.1 Mobilizing Structure ... 63
3.3.2 Sequential Targeting ... 66
3.3.3 Make a Scene: Open Art of Resistance ... 68
3.4 Safe Hospital Project and Selective Punishment ... 70
3.4.1 Background ... 70
3.4.2 Selective Punishment and Its Rationale ... 72
3.4.3 Self-protection Strategies of Hospitals ... 78
3.5 Summary ... 81
References ... 82

4 The Art of Persuasion: Everyday Mediation Practice ... 85
4.1 Introduction ... 86
4.1.1 Standard Operation in Dispute Mediation ... 88
4.2 Mediation Channel: Breaking the Power Asymmetry ... 90
4.3 The Art of Mediation ... 95
4.3.1 Dynamic Goals and Toolkit of Mediators ... 95
4.3.2 Politicization ... 95
4.3.3 Affective Strategy ... 99
4.3.4 Compensation Bargaining ... 103
4.4 Summary ... 108
References ... 110

5 From Right Protection to Monetary Bargaining ... 113
5.1 Money Matters: Bargained Authoritarianism ... 114
5.2 Rationale in Compensation Distribution ... 118
5.2.1 Framework of Rationale for Compensation Distribution ... 118
5.2.2 In Quest for Distributive Justice ... 119
5.2.3 Political Stability—Discretion to Troublemakers ... 120
5.2.4 Economic Cost Concerns ... 121
5.2.5 Where Does the Money Come from? ... 122
5.2.6 Data and Variables ... 124
5.3 Findings ... 125
5.3.1 Empirical Results ... 127
5.3.2 Qualitative Evidence: Buying Stability for ALL? ... 130
5.4 The Limits of Bargained Authoritarianism ... 138
5.5 Summary ... 140
References ... 142

6 Conclusion ... 145
6.1 Overview ... 145
6.2 Patients, Doctors, and Mediators ... 147
6.3 Politicized Social Disputes Resolution ... 152

6.4 Bargaining-Style Mediation 154
6.5 Implications and Limitations of the Study 157
References 162

Appendix A: List of Interview and Interview Script 165

Appendix B 169

Appendix C: Glossary of Chinese Terms 171

About the Author

Dr. Jie Wu (吴洁) is an assistant professor of the political science department at Fudan University. She received Ph.D. from the University of Hong Kong. She obtained her B.A. and M.A. (Political Science) degrees from Fudan University. Her research interests revolve around health policy, contentious politics, and state-society relations in China. Her prior research and study were supported by the Swire Scholarship and Harvard-Yenching Institute. Her studies have appeared in *The China Journal*, *China Information*, *International Public Management Review*, *CJPS*, *China Review*, etc.

Chapter 1
Introduction

City—Before dawn, *Doctor Jiang* received a night call from the hospital to perform an emergency operation for a heart attack patient, the second emergency call he had received that night. An hour later, he posted a line on social media:

> A perfect day from 7 am to 10 pm, and then from 2 to 6 am.

Then, he took a quick shower and returned to the office for another day-long shift.

XiaoJiang (little Jiang), a freshly graduated nurse dispatched to the psychiatry department for her internship, cried silently in the office because a patient with a mental disorder had beaten her for no reason.

Doctor Wei put on a shield and took a selfie that he posted online, making fun of the insecure working environment of doctors in public hospitals. It aroused heated discussion online and was reposted by many netizens. A few minutes later, he was asked by his supervisor to delete the post and apologize for creating a tense atmosphere between doctors and patients that could endanger the image of a harmonious society.

Hospitial security Guard Zhu, a man in his late 40s, wore his uniform and stood in front of the emergency room to prevent anxious family members from interrupting treatment. Young nurses greeted him by making jokes about him, creating an atmosphere interweaving both tension and casualness.

Mr. Chen, a migrant farmer who lived in a rural part of the city, took his child to a renowned children's hospital. After waiting over four hours before receiving treatment from the doctor, his son died. In an open letter to the head of the hospital, he expressed his discontentment about the indifference shown by the doctors and nurses who let his son die without adequate and efficient treatment. He asked for a public apology and compensation for all the expenses of raising a child. He wrote (Fig. 1.1):

> Dear Chief representative of the Hospital (院长),
>
> My wife is disabled and experienced dangerous bleeding when giving birth to my son. My two-year-old son was sent to the hospital at 14:40, and it was not until 19:00 that the hospital

J. Wu, *Politicized Medical Dispute Resolution in China*, Understanding China,
https://doi.org/10.1007/978-981-97-6961-2_1

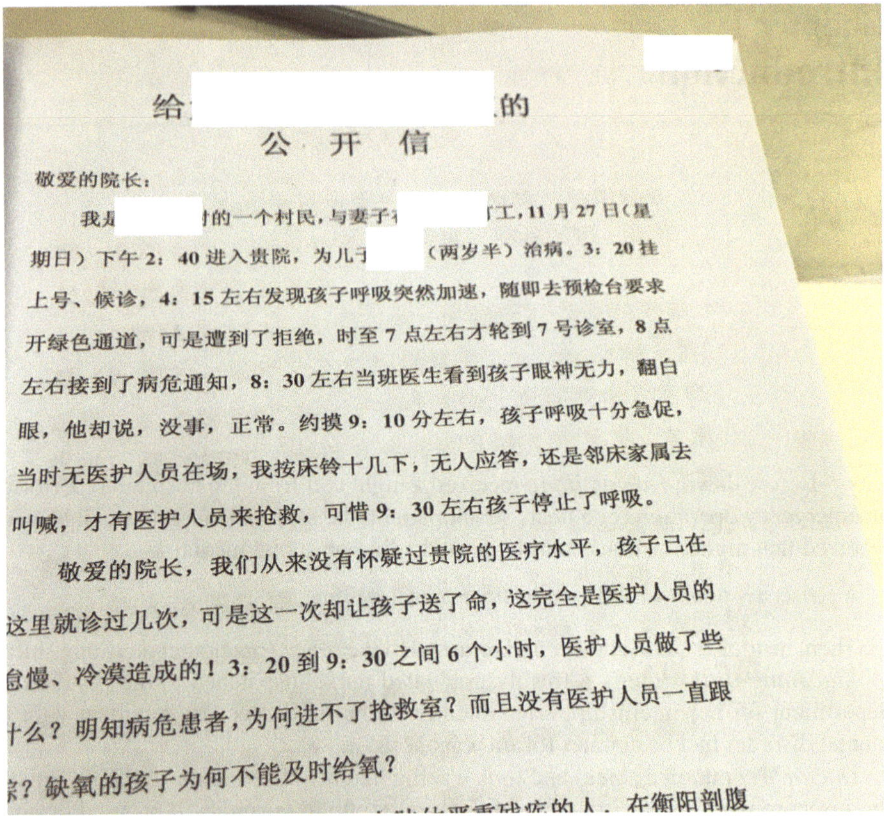

给[redacted]的
公 开 信

敬爱的院长：

我是[redacted]村的一个村民，与妻子在[redacted]打工，11月27日(星期日）下午2：40进入贵院，为儿子[redacted]（两岁半）治病。3：20挂上号、候诊，4：15左右发现孩子呼吸突然加速，随即去预检台要求开绿色通道，可是遭到了拒绝，时至7点左右才轮到7号诊室，8点左右接到了病危通知，8：30左右当班医生看到孩子眼神无力，翻白眼，他却说，没事，正常。约摸9：10分左右，孩子呼吸十分急促，当时无医护人员在场，我按床铃十几下，无人应答，还是邻床家属去叫喊，才有医护人员来抢救，可惜9：30左右孩子停止了呼吸。

敬爱的院长，我们从来没有怀疑过贵院的医疗水平，孩子已在这里就诊过几次，可是这一次却让孩子送了命，这完全是医护人员的怠慢、冷漠造成的！3：20到9：30之间6个小时，医护人员做了些什么？明知病危患者，为何进不了抢救室？而且没有医护人员一直跟踪？缺氧的孩子为何不能及时给氧？

Fig. 1.1 Open letter from the patient family. *Source* Archived from the fieldwork

> admitted him after waiting for nearly five hours. His situation worsened at eight o'clock in the evening, yet the doctor did not provide any effective treatment. He began to show shortness of breath at 21:10 and died at 21:30 after the first aid. The purpose of this open letter is not for money but just to find justice for my poor son (讨公道).[1]

Police Officer Zhang, a retired police officer, had experience dealing with all kinds of street-level confrontations, including family and neighbourhood disputes. His jurisdiction covered several major district hospitals that attracted thousands of patients nationwide. He had good relations with the healthcare professionals and hospital representatives and, after retirement, was hired as a part-time mediator to address medical disputes between patients and the involved hospitals in his district. His daily job is to address the medical disputes between patients and hospitals within the jurisdiction, prevent hospital violence, and maintain social order.

The lives of a migrant farmer, a former police officer, and different types of medical professionals are connected through the hospital. Neither the healthcare

[1] Based on the fieldwork data on September 2016.

professionals nor the patients are satisfied with their situation, with all parties considering themselves "victims" of the system. This has turned hospitals into powder kegs. Nowadays, hospitals, which reflect the lives and deaths of ordinary Chinese citizens, have become the focal point of conflicts. In a health system designed to support a population of over 1.4 billion, discontent and hospital violence deteriorate patient-doctor trust, hinder high-quality health service provision, endanger social stability, and create troubles for contemporary China's rulers and governments.

1.1 Puzzle

Patient-doctor relations are experiencing a crisis in China. Mistrust between doctors and patients (Chan, 2018) coupled with unaffordable health care (Yip et al., 2010) and hospital corruption scandals (Chan & Yao, 2018) have led to increasing tension between patients and doctors. Coinciding with Chinese citizens' rising consciousness of rights and law (Gallagher, 2006; Li, 2010; Pan, 2002; Perry, 2009), patients are increasingly suing doctors for medical malpractice or unsatisfactory medical service (He, 2014; He & Qian, 2016). Pushed to the limits, some have turned to collective action or even violence to assert their rights (Liebman, 2013; Xu, 2014), readdress their grievances, or simply "eye-for-eye" justice. According to a 2006 survey by the China Hospital Management Association, over 70% of China's public hospitals have experienced hospital violence (Zhao et al., 2018), with patients acting violently toward medical workers to express anger, protect their rights, or for monetary reasons. According to the National Health and Planning Committee, there were over 1,007,000 medical disputes in China in 2016, including 4,037 cases that involved violent behavior towards healthcare professionals.[2] Increased hospital violence incidents and medical disputes have been widely reported and touched the nerves of Chinese governments, who must balance responding to vulnerable patients' claims to show their moral responsibility with maintaining social order and stability in public spaces.

What drives patients to adopt hospital violence as an extreme measure in China's constrained political space? What turns medical disputes between patients and doctors into social conflicts between citizens and government authorities? Why and how does the government intervene in medical disputes? This book touches upon an interesting and important topic, medical disputes, including their violent form—hospital violence (also known as medical disturbance). Drawing on two years of intensive fieldwork, this book analyzes patients' strategies and presents how citizens adopt non-compliance behaviors to hold public hospitals and the government accountable, given China's tightened political constraints. More crucially, it argues that medical dispute resolution has been politicized, its process and outcomes shaped

[2] See, for instance, There were 100,700 medical disputes nationwide in 2016. How should the doctor-patient relationship be resolved? https://www.chinairn.com/news/20170309/15295954.shtml, accessed on September 11, 2023.

by multiple influencing factors, including legal regulations and rules, moral norms, and political concerns. Burdened by conflicting goals, the medical dispute resolution process has also become a political bargaining process between patients, hospitals, and government agents. The politicization of medical disputes addresses stability maintenance concerns but may commercialize patient-doctor relations, erode social trust, and endanger the rule of law. This book joins the debate about contentious Chinese politics and examines the interaction between the government and its citizens, while examining medical disputes from a social science perspective.

Why do patients resort to hospital violence? Organizing contentious misbehavior or creating disturbances is highly risky in China and likely to result in government repression. Studies on contentious politics have analyzed China's political opportunity structure and explained the relationship between protesters' strategies and dynamic government responses (Cai, 2008; 2020; Chen, 2012; 2020; Li et al., 2012; Lorentzen, 2017). Although the literature offers many insights, few examine the occurrence of hospital violence from the perspective of rightful resistance and the government's response strategies.

The uniqueness of medical disputes lies in two aspects. On the one hand, hospital violence could be considered non-compliance behavior—a law-breaking but not regime-threatening action intended to evoke government responses to address citizens' grievances (Tsai, 2015). Unlike rightful resistance organized by peasants and labor organizations, medical disputes target non-government institutions and are thus less regime-threatening, sustaining their occurrence in China's limited political space. On the other hand, the nature of medical dispute has also prompted scholars to rethink the moral perspective in collective actions that limit the government's latitude to employ repressive measures. Eric Hobsbawm (1974) developed the "social bandit" concept to explain the psychological perspective of the rise of proletarian protest against an exploitative elite class. The concept shifts scholars' focus to the moral capital the powerless hold in collective actions. Patients' embedded moral power and quest for rights are intertwined in medical disputes, with tragedy and pain justifying their contentious and sometimes irrational behavior against authorities. Patients in China are often depicted as vulnerable, weak, and needing assistance to arouse public sympathy, which equips them with natural moral power in bargaining with the state, staying officials from resorting to repression (Leung & Nann, 1995). Having only the power of the weak (Scott, 1985), patients are unlikely to be viewed as strong opponents or rivals by the socialist regime. Harsh repression towards the weakness often conflicts with the moral image of the benevolent state, tying the rulers' hands in regulating noncompliance behaviors. This weakness encourages the regime to deploy novel, multifaceted response strategies, and concession or leniency often results. This book speaks to the moral perspective of collective actions in China using hospital violence as a case study.

This book theorizes China's politicized civil dispute resolution process, which directly touches the lives of patients and healthcare professionals. As contentious behaviors have become "normalized" or "routinized" (Perry & Selden, 2000; Chen, 2012), China's government has become more sophisticated in dealing with these bottom-up collective actions. Rather than using direct repression and cooptation to maintain regime stability in dealing with social disputes that do not directly target the regime, Chinese authorities have revitalized and institutionalized semi-legal mediation channels to settle social disputes and absorb grievances (Fan, 2000; Hu, 2011; Minzner, 2011; Zhang & Cai, 2019; Zhuang & Chen, 2015). It relies on semi-government officials to act as mediators and become the intermediary between citizens and public institutions, remaking what Philip Huang (1993) called "the third realm" in contemporary China. The strategy seeks to resolve potential collective actions before they can occur, as a form of preventive and "covert" repression (Davenport, 2005; Earl, 2003; 2011). This book examines the institutional adaptation of mediation institutions from the Mao era to today and how it has been refashioned to address emerging social disputes. This book documents strategic and complex interactions between patients, healthcare professionals, and mediators in medical dispute resolution. It investigates a series of deterring, affective, and bargaining strategies that mediators, as semi-government officials, employ to balance hospital and patient interests. It looks deeper into the daily interactions between citizens and the government in addressing their disputes in China.

Moreover, this book also examines the "buying stability" strategy (花钱买平安) routinely applied in China. When attempting to resolve social disputes, citizens commonly target local governments, holding them accountable for addressing their monetary claims. Governments sometimes pay much more money than necessary in exchange for "peace" or to silence the disputant, termed "buying stability" (Lee & Zhang, 2013; Benney, 2016). However, it may unexpectedly encourage the spread of contentious tactics by providing economic incentives towards disruptive actions and increasing the economic cost burden among local governments. Although monetary compensation has become a significant approach to dealing with bottom-up social grievances (Lee & Zhang, 2013), few studies examine the compensation distribution rationale and the efficacy of the disputants' strategies in shaping the outcomes. This book traces the intricate rationale in government compensation distribution and examines the government's strategic objectives embedded in dispute resolution using medical disputes as a case. Unlike in other social disputes, putting a price on human life seems unacceptable when addressing medical disputes (Zelizer, 2017; 2018). However, in China, monetary compensation distribution seems still a key approach to addressing grievances in medical dispute resolution. This book aims to unveil the compensation distribution mechanism for redressing social disputes by drawing on empirical data on medical disputes and weighting such factors as legal rules, public perceptions of justice, and political considerations. By assessing compensation distribution, this book examines citizens' efficacy in bargaining with the government and explains how China succeeds in shifting citizens' focus from rights protection to economic benefits to restore the social order.

Neither hospital violence nor medical disputes are unique to China. They also occur in other national and regional settings, such as India, Israel, and Russia (Kumar et al., 2016). However, due to the state's strong embeddedness in Chinese society, a single problem can escalate into a larger picture and politicize specific social and political problems. For instance, since public hospitals—which account for eighty per cent of healthcare resources—are funded by the Chinese government, Chinese citizens often shifted their blame from the public institution to the entire healthcare system and local government. In a similar vein, as Lei and Zhou (2015) found in cases of public opinion towards food safety scandals in China, netizens concluded that the "Sanlu milk scandal [was] ultimately rooted in [the] political regime (p. 581)." The pan-political responsibility attribution process prompted the government's intervention to regulate the social relations between public institutions and citizens. The political embeddedness of the health system made the government's responsibility for and intervention in social dispute resolution inevitable. Failing to be responsive to social grievances may endanger the regime's moral legitimacy.

It is never easy to address medical disputes. Governments must make constant trade-offs between professional groups and citizens. However, in China, over sixty per cent of medical disputes have been channeled to mediation institutions, with success rates as high as 85 per cent.[3] What explains this success? How was it achieved? In this book, I examine the lessons and outcomes and the policy implications of this trade-off between citizens and hospitals. Therefore, using medical dispute cases as a thread, this book takes readers into the dark box of dispute resolution and state-society interactions in China.

1.2 Political Participation and Institutional Responses in China

> Authoritarian regimes are characterized by the lack of political opportunities for collective action, but this does not mean that popular resistance is absent in such regimes. (Cai, 2008).

China's rapid social and economic development has given rise to all types of disputes, ranging from interest-related conflicts, such as land and labor disputes, to interpersonal disputes, including family and neighborhood conflicts. When bottom-up disputes are not addressed promptly, they often evolve into protests or collective actions that create social disturbances and erode social stability in rural and urban settings. It has been over 30 years since China's popular contention became a field of scholarly interest. With the rapid growth of publications on contentious politics in China, questions remain on how the theories could interpret acts of bottom-up popular resistance and the state's diverse coping strategies.

The question of popular contention has captured scholarly attention for understanding non-electoral political participation in China. Building on their deep concern, O'Brien and Li Lianjiang (2006) conceptualized the popular contention adopted in peasant petitions as "rightful resistance", entailing the tactical use of law, policies, and other officially endorsed values to punish corrupt cadres and protect their interests (O'Brien, 1996, p. 33). They suggest that peasants in rural China take

[3] See, for instance, More than 60% of medical disputes in China are resolved through people's mediation, with a success rate of 85%, http://www.xinhuanet.com/politics/2019-02/15/c_1124116833.htm, accessed on September 13, 2023.

actions between institutionalized participation and popular resistance to pressure local governments while avoiding political red lines, showing their "nascent rights consciousness (Li, 2010, p. 2)".

Beyond rural settings, scholars have focused on the various tactics and strategies different social classes apply to achieve their goals; for instance, Cai Yongshun's studies on middle-class residents in urban settings (Cai, 2005) and laid-off workers in North China's rust-belt region (Cai, 2002), Lee's (2007) study on new merging workers in South China, and Diamant and O'Brien's (2015) and Yang's (2022) studies on veterans' compensation issues. Scholars have provided very detailed summaries of how individuals take action to negotiate with the state and their different outcomes. Various social classes have mobilized to achieve their aims or obtain written rights through political participation to prioritize their pursuits, protect their personal or collective interests, and seek the state's benevolence. However, different social classes' varying resources, strategies, and mobilization capabilities have led to their collective actions having different outcomes. For instance, Table 1.1 summarizes the characteristics of citizens in addressing different issues, drawing from the literature on contentious politics.

Though the rise of popular contention has made it challenging for local governments to maintain stability and the incentives to avoid skip-level petitions, it is "far less politically threatening" from a political perspective (Perry, 2008, p. 29). Rightful resistance is still a within-system form of contention that operates in the reform paradigm, not the revolution paradigm (O'Brien, 2013, p. 17), and rarely clashes with state authority (Perry, 2008). On the one hand, citizens mainly focus on personal or group-based interests, rarely on public or rights-related ones (Chen, 2020). A few exceptions are rights-related advocacy, such as feminist protests, that may lead to

Table 1.1 Studies of various types of social disputes in China

Issue	Protesters	Author
Compensation	Laid-off workers	Cai (2002)
		Chen (2003)
	Retired/laid-off	Blecher (2002)
	Migrant workers	Lee (2007)
	Veterans	Diamant and O'Brien (2015) and Yang (2022)
Land/real estate disputes	Peasants	Li (2006)
	Urban middle class	(Cai 2005)
		Shi and Cai (2006) Sheng (2017)
	Hui Muslim Community	Luo and Andreas (2016)
Environment	Urban middle class	Zhong and Hwang (2016)
Policy failure/social injustice	Peasants	O'Brien and Li (2006)
		Hurst et al. (2014)

repression.[4] In other words, the nature of rightful resistance was sometimes disguised by the name "right" despite involving core material and personal interests. On the other hand, citizens are often carefully framed to proactively align with the state's rhetoric and avoid pinpointing structural and institutional problems. For instance, Kuang and Göbel's (2013) study confirmed how citizens carefully chose Maoist narratives that gave meaning to their collective actions and resonated with state-confirmed rhetoric. Their bottom-up resistance remained parochial, often confined to one region, targeting local government (O'Brien, 2002; Yang, 2023) rather than the central government to constrain their regime-threatening nature. Citizens could strategically apply popular contention to shape local government's policy agenda or prioritize their demands.

To address increased political participation while acknowledging the non-regime-threatening nature of rightful resistance, the government redirects citizens to institutionalized channels to address their grievances and popular discontent instead of resorting to direct repression. According to Pepinsky (2013; 2014), under authoritarianism, elites purposefully create institutions that consolidate their hold on political power to foster durable rule. To achieve legitimacy and maintain social order, rulers need to maintain social stability and show responsiveness to the citizens' grievances simultaneously. The government has revitalized, created, or adapted a series of institutional channels in contemporary China to absorb the bottom-up grievance and maintain social stability. This book examines the effect of mediation institutions on dispute resolution.

First, since the reform and opening up, the post-Mao Chinese government has prioritized rule-by-law to build its legitimacy and address social disputes. A series of laws have been promulgated, including the Administrative Procedure Law (1989)[5] and Organic Law of Villagers' Committees (1987),[6] to regulate the relations between citizens, public institutions, and government. The Party-state has deliberatively mobilized law or cultivated "law consciousness" to encourage and redirect citizens to use law instrumentally to address their social and civil disputes. However, Chinese disputants' increasing "law consciousness" can backfire.

On the one hand, political scholars find that accommodating democracy by implementing "Organic Law" at the grassroots level is not always easy in a one-party state. It may mobilize citizens by providing them with the grounds for resistance and political participation, which could weaken the Party's rule at the grassroots level (e.g., see O'Brien & Li, 2000). On the other hand, legal scholars find that law consciousness and mobilization have led to a litigation explosion, with unprecedented numbers of cases being filed in courts (Fan, 2000). However, the law cannot depict itself as "[a] capable protector", as it fails to address the problems that led to the civil disputes and preserve citizens' rights. For instance, Chen's (2004) study shows that, frequently,

[4] For instance, see Fu & Distelhorst (2018).

[5] See, for instance, Administrative Litigation Law of the People's Republic of China, https://www.gov.cn/flfg/2006-10/29/content_1499268.htm, accessed on September 12, 2023.

[6] See, for instance, Organic Law of the Villagers' Committees of the People's Republic of China, http://www.reformdata.org/1987/1124/7754.shtml, accessed on September 12, 2023.

neither party is satisfied with the results of a trial: the prevailing party often complains about ineffective law enforcement, which makes the verdict a rubber stamp, while the losing party often attributes their failure to injustice in the system and the low quality of legal workers, threatening to petition a higher-level court for relief. Some repeat petitioners often threatened to adopt disruptive behaviors to prioritize their pursuits. Hence, legal workers are vulnerable to popular will, media pressure, protesters, and violence (Liebman, 2007; 2013; 2015; Fu, 2015), making court a heavy burden, dampening the authority of legal institutions, and forcing them to bow to popular pressure. More crucially, the legal channels—courts—must balance the sometimes conflicting goals of upholding justice and maintaining social stability, further destabilizing the regime (Minzner, 2011; Liebman, 2017; Ng & He, 2017). The half-hearted rule of law has undermined rather than enhanced social stability, exposing China's weak institutional environment. As Gallagher (2017) contended, the instrumental use of the law has brought dysfunction, unintentionally exposed the weak efficacy of legal institutions, and encouraged more bottom-up popular resistance.

Given the inefficacy of formal legal channels, extra-legal bureaucratic mechanisms were revitalized as institutional bricolage, adapting traditional institutions for new goals in a process Carl Minzner (2011) called retreating from the rule of law. Among these mechanisms, the Letter and Visit Bureau (*xinfang*, 信访) has received the most scholarly attention. From the Party's establishment, Mao Zedong encouraged people to use letters and visits to express their opinions towards the Party. For instance, in 1921, two workers from colliery wrote to Mao, suggesting he should care about the labor movement as he had the peasant movement.[7] Mao attached great importance to the letter and went to Anyuan in person, an act later known as the roots of the Party-state's revolutionary tradition (Perry, 2012). It strengthened Mao's belief in the importance of the letter and visit system. As Mao stated on July 14, 1941 (Mao, 1996, Volume 3, p. 189)

> (W)e need pay great attention to listen to the opinions from the people ... through all types of conferences, newspapers, letters and calls, we can always find their true voices.

This tradition persisted after the establishment of China in 1949, following the mass-line strategy. In 1954, all central government ministries and departments established letter and visit bureaus staffed by full- and part-time cadres (Chen, 2004). This practice diffused across local government, achieving graduated management by department and level. Different from legal channels, it reflected the Party-state's mass-line strategy of responding directly to suggestions, connections, and complaints from the people through bureaucratic absorption. From the central government perspective, this enhanced the regime's information capability to discipline an incapable bureaucracy, improved governance, and won the hearts of the masses, enhancing grassroots power. From the bottom-up perspective, it was an effective channel for citizens to express their grievances and address their civil disputes, especially those with the local government (Minzner, 2006).

---

[7] See, for instance, Gao Wuping: On the preservation and abolition of the petition system - and on the reform of China's petition syste, https://www.aisixiang.com/data/5827.html, accessed on May 18, 2024.

Despite disappearing during the turbulent Cultural Revolution, the Letter and Visit Bureau was revived in the reform and open-up era. The 1982 Constitution of the People's Republic of China stated, "Chinese citizens have the right to criticize and make suggestions to any state agency and public personnel"[8] (Constitution, 1982, article 41). Since the reform and opening up, *xinfang* institutions have experienced more frequent visits than ever due to the changing social and political lives. The main theme of public claims has shifted from political to economic ones, such as urban demolition, compensation-related pursuits, or complaints about heavy tax burdens. Meanwhile, citizens' modes of participation have also become more intense and violent (Fang, 2009). To curb violence during the *xinfang*, the Regulation on Letter and Visits, passed in 2005, regulated troublemaking behavior by forbidding citizens from holding illegal gatherings, attacking state agencies, or blocking traffic (Article 20).[9] As the flow of petitions, range of grievances, and level of anger mounted, institutions gradually became bureaucratized to absorb the grievances and become a tool for social stability. As Feng Shizheng (2012) commented, since the reform and opening up, the main goal of the *xinfang* institution has not been to mobilize the masses to find and manufacture social antagonism but to facilitate social integration to resolve social conflicts and maintain social stability.

The efficacy of *xinfang* institution remains controversial. Many scholars have acknowledged their crucial role in enhancing autocratic duality by exercising social control to maintain social stability (Wang & Minzner, 2015), enhancing the rulers' information collection capacity (Huang et al., 2019), and showing responsiveness to citizens by selectively respond to their appeals (Meng et al., 2017). As a result, mounting collective actions did not lead to regime change (Dimitrov, 2008; Lorentzen, 2013) but enhanced the state's capacity to cope with social unrest.

Other scholars assert that *xinfang* institutions, which mainly rely on bureaucratic rules, still have boundaries. Chen Xi (2012) found that such quasi-democratic institutions have unexpectedly contributed to the rise of collective behaviors. The Letter and Visit Bureau tried to absorb a "laundry list" of complaints and selectively responded to address grievances, especially those that can arouse collective actions. The government's appliance of concession has made troublemaking tactics an attractive way for protestors to have their demands prioritized. For instance, the local state, pressured by citizens' skip-level petitioning, often offered concessions in exchange for inactivity. Greg Distelhorst (2017) found that activists exploit the same institutions to seek concessions from agencies and realize their demands. Sometimes, repetitive petitioners were somewhat trapped by the "bureaucratization" in *xinfang* institutions. The Letter and Visit Bureau's low efficacy and failure to address grievances has led to collective actions. Hence, at the beginning of the 2000s, Yu (2005; 2016) suggested abolishing the *xinfang* system as it may channel bottom-up grievances to

[8] See, for instance, Constitution of the People's Republic of China (1982), http://www.npc.gov.cn/zgrdw/npc/zt/qt/gjxfz/2014-12/03/content_1888093.htm, accessed on September 13, 2023.

[9] See, for instance, Decree of the State Council of the People's Republic of China: Regulations on Letters and Visits, https://www.gov.cn/gongbao/content/2005/content_63338.htm, accessed on September 15, 2023.

the central government, endangering the regime's legitimacy, and fuel activism and collective actions; additionally, a lack of institutional professionalism may dampen the legitimacy of legal institutions. However, the idea has encountered bureaucratic and scholarly opposition for blocking existing limited citizens' interest representation channels, especially for the powerless and the vulnerable.

Realizing the shortcomings in the courts and *xinfang* institutions, the Chinese government shifted from legal and bureaucratic approaches to more integrated and pragmatic attitudes in addressing social disputes. In recent years, we have witnessed the revival of an old-yet-new political institution—People's Mediation—that combines legal professionalism and mass-line ideology in dispute resolution. Since President Xi Jinping took office, many institutions that trace back to the Mao era have been institutionalized and revived as institutional bricolage (Koss, 2021) to address emerging social and political governance issues.

This book examines People's Mediation Institutions (*renmin tiaojie*, or mediation) embedded with legal, political, and social power for dispute resolution. The adaptiveness and uniqueness of mediation channels are three-fold. First, China's People's Mediation institution functions as an alternative dispute resolution channel, yet still based on laws and regulations. Second, the institution bears political responsibility to balance the interests of individuals and groups, maintain social stability, and prevent social disputes from escalating. Third, in a tradition inherited from the Imperia era, the institution relies on a new "social gentry"—politically embedded mediators—to address disputes and rebuild social power. By channeling citizens into a mediation channel, it aims to ease the caseloads of the courts and government bureaus, maintain harmonious relations between the disputants, and rebuild grassroots social order through the mediators' intermediary role.

In this book, I examine the institutional change of People's Mediation and investigate its efficacy in absorbing discontent in addressing social disputes. The People's Mediation channels are not only channels to address disputes but also vehicles for distributing monetary compensation and resources to enhance regime durability. Mediation institutions allow for state intervention, permit citizens' expression of grievance as a social safety valve, and enable monetary distribution to settle social disputes. Mediation institutions mainly deal with compensation-related and materialistic-involved disputes. The non-regime-threatening nature of their claims provides the political opportunity structure for citizens to exert rightful resistance to realize their interests. In dealing with these social disputes, the Chinese government relies on the mediation channel to achieve complex goals, including satisfying the popular perception of redistributive justice, maintaining political stability, and rebuilding social power. This book investigates the politicization process of social dispute resolution through mediation institutions and its unintended consequences.

This book examines the occurrence of medical disputes, including their violent form—hospital violence and institutional responses from the government in China. It dialogues with various streams of literature, from political science and China studies to sociology and health policy, crossing disciplines to explain why hospital violence occurs in China and the government's strategies for addressing its citizens' grievances. Instead of viewing hospital violence as a type of individual or collective violence, the author examines the occurrence of hospital disturbances from the political participation perspective, which reflects another facet of non-electoral political participation in China.

Chinese citizens increasingly use political behaviors to negotiate with the state to realize their interests and solve disputes. Returning to rightful resistance theory, O'Brien and Li (2006) suggested that rural citizens muddle institutionalized participation and popular resistance to achieve their interests (O'Brien, 1996, p. 33). Today, Chinese citizens carefully frame their grievances and discontent to realize their written rights and interests through various modes of mobilization and protest tactics. Chen Xi (2009, 2012) further categorizes and labels them as the power of "troublemaking" (*nao*, 闹), defined as petitioners' disruptive tactics, which could gain high efficacy. This book examines hospital violence as a less contentious form of political participation in health institutions and examines the varied and changing government responses towards hospital violence.

Second, this book empirically examines how and why medical disputes have been politized through mediation institutions in China. The medical dispute resolution this book describes directly touches the lives of patients and healthcare professionals in contemporary China. This book theorizes the politicalized civil dispute resolution process in China. In addition to using direct repression and cooptation to maintain regime stability, Chinese authorities have institutionalized semi-legal mediation channels to settle social disputes. It seeks to resolve potential collective actions before they have the chance to take place, as a form of preventive repression. This book documents strategic and complex interactions between patients, healthcare professionals, and mediators in medical dispute resolution. It investigates a series of deterring, affective, and bargaining strategies the government employs in the mediation process to transform medical disputes from rights protection to monetary bargaining and balance hospital and patient interests. It looks deeper into the daily interactions between citizens and the government in addressing their disputes in China.

Mediation institution is an increasingly important part of authoritarian institutions to absorb bottom-up grievances. Most scholarly attention on mediation has focused on labor or land disputes, which have a high possibility of leading to collective actions or civic disputes between citizens and local government (e.g., Zhuang & Chen, 2015; Chen, 2003); few have examined medical disputes, which involve professional knowledge, heightened emotion, and less-contentious forms of political participation. In most cities, specific people's mediation institutions for medical disputes have recently been widely established with the increasing caseload growth. Medical dispute resolution cannot be handled merely by legal rules; social rules and political priority also play major roles in medical disputes' outcomes and decisions. This book examines the institutional boundaries of the mediation channel and its multiple institutional logic, which jointly shape the dispute resolution process, outcome, and efficacy.

Third, this book adds a new, political perspective to existing studies examining the doctor-patient relationship in China. It examines the institutional constraints of hospitals and healthcare professionals in contemporary China and how they jointly shape the politicized dispute resolution's outcomes and process. It reconsiders medical disputes beyond the medical perspective to disclose the largely behind-the-scenes struggles between patients, doctors, and mediators. In the medical dispute resolution process, the visible and inimitable power of politics has, to some extent, shaped doctor-patient relations to maintain social order and a harmonious society.

1.3 Background: A Brief Historical Account of the Chinese Health System

The Chinese health system's history reflects China's ideological changes and evolving governance model. Since the Republic of China, professional elites and the government have promoted state medicine compatible with the modern state's responsibility to provide health services nationwide in rural and urban settings. Unfortunately, the system was neither satisfactory nor universal due to political and financial limitations (Gao, 2012). When the Communist Party of China came into power in 1949, the traditional Chinese health system was reorganized in a "command and control" manner (Eggleston et al., 2008; Wagstaff et al., 2009). Prior, eighty per cent of the doctors in China practiced medicine autonomously and privately or were organized by medical associations (Zhou, 2020; Yao, 2015, p. 54). Since 1949, the whole health system has been financed by the state and organized around the work unit or "*danwei*", and most healthcare professionals have been reorganized and nationalized, becoming state or public employees (Henderson & Cohen, 1984). With the removal of medical professional associations, healthcare professionals lost the bargaining power to negotiate with the state (Davis, 2000; Yao, 2015). The hospital was both a professional institution and an important public organ like other Soviet-style institutions (Lampton, 1977). Healthcare professionals became public employees deeply embedded within the political personnel system. They were considered important components of the cadre system with special expertise and enjoying a monthly allowance that reflected their prestige as state functionaries rather than autonomous professionals (Field, 1991; Freidson, 1984). This bred tension between professionals and the state in the following decades.

The health system was structured as a hierarchy that relied on the professional authority mechanism. Professional norms inevitably conflicted with the Party-state's ideological pursuits. Under expert logic, professionals pursued advancement and innovation in the health field. For instance, most advanced health institutions were concentrated in large cities, while secondary-level care was provided in township health centers and urban district or enterprise hospitals (Wagstaff et al., 2009), leaving rural areas less covered and health resources scarce and causing uneven distribution of high-quality healthcare resources between urban and rural areas, contrary to equality-based communist ideology. Health problems including famine, epidemic disease, and child malnutrition have heavily struck the rural areas, which dampened agricultural production and the authority of the Party (Zhou, 2017). The primary health delivery was inefficient, selective, and scarce. Mao blamed health authority leaders for prioritizing urban development and ignoring rural areas in a speech on June 26th, 1965 (known as the 626 talk):

> The Ministry of Public Health is not a Ministry of Public Health for the people, so why not change its name to the Ministry of Urban Health, the Ministry of Gentlemen's Health, or even to the Ministry of Urban Gentlemen's (*laoye*, 老爷) Health? (Schram & Chinnery, 1974; p. 232).

Driven by ideology, the focus of the health care system in the 1960s shifted from urban areas and high-cutting medical technologies to a preventive public health scheme and rural areas to improve national health provision. In order to boost the supply of medical workers nationwide by a giant leap, radical changes took place, converging the Soviet model and innovative indigenous measures through mass mobilization. First, Mao downplayed the role of the "professional" while emphasizing practical knowledge and preventive medicine. Many doctors (nearly one-third of the staff in urban areas) needed to rotate from urban to rural areas as reeducation to address villagers' health issues (Chen, 2001). Mao promoted shortening the medical education curriculum and sent students to the countryside to sharpen their techniques. The supervision and management of medical training were also decentralized by allowing regional variances; governments could customize curricula based on local resources and conditions. As Mao stated,

> Medical education should be reformed. There is no need to read so many books. How many years did Hua Tuo (a famous ancient Chinese physician) spend at college? … It will be enough to give three years to graduates from higher primary schools. They would then study and raise their standards mainly through practice" (Schram & Chinnery, 1974, p. 233).

Meanwhile, to reinforce Mao's notion of equality and provide accessible and affordable care to rural areas, Barefoot Doctor schemes (*chi jiao yisheng*, 赤脚医生) were launched in rural areas to prevent disease and publicize basic medical information under a mass campaign (Sidel, 1972). A barefoot doctor was half peasant and half medical worker, receiving three to six months of introductory medical training and practices in Chinese traditional medicine and acupuncture before being sent to rural areas to deliver primary health services (Wang, 1975).

The goal of the health reform was to improve the health provision in rural areas in a cost-efficient manner through mass mobilization. During this time, Chinese traditional medicine, as a symbolic token of indigenous traditional wisdom, was integrated with Western medicine to make medicine less costly and more accessible and promote a sense of national pride. Meanwhile, many rural areas adopted rural cooperation schemes to improve the health service provision, funded by local people's communes (Chen, 2001; Wang, 2009). Under its "prevention first strategy", rural cooperative medicine schemes, with the help of grassroots barefoot doctors, provided villagers with cheaper, accessible medicine and mobilized rural residents to improve their health conditions and living environments.

Mao's downplaying of professionals and experts doubtless hindered the professional development of medical knowledge and professional autonomy. On the other hand, however, public healthcare was provided at a lower cost and greatly improved in rural areas, despite political disturbances. Many scholars worldwide have praised the barefoot doctor model's cost-efficiency, calling it a role model for developing countries with limited resources to improve health coverage and conditions. The life expectancy of Chinese citizens greatly improved from 1949 to 1981, climbing from 35 years to 67.8.[10] Yet, great success was achieved through mass mobilization and government decentralization, which was enabled by the then collective economic and agriculture system in rural China.

In Deng Xiaoping's era, the overall governance model shifted from a planned to a market-based economy to free the government from direct involvement in managing the public sector. The introduction of market-oriented reform changed the health system landscape. In a larger picture, the central government gradually retrenched and decentralized its power over and financial support for the healthcare system (Hsiao, 1995), with the local governments now shouldering financial responsibility for health services in their region. The varied pace of economic and social development across the country led to a fragmented health system.

The changing government model made public hospitals fragile and exposed them to the market environment. On the supply side, the retrenchment of government funding created economic incentives for hospitals to profit independently, transferring public hospitals from work units to semi-for-profit organizations. According to Ministry of Health (MOH) statistics, direct government subsidies accounted for less than 10.81% of hospitals' total revenue in 1987, compared to 23.87% in 1980 (Zhang, 1999). To compensate for shrinking subsidies, the government decentralized its power and "allowed" hospitals more autonomy to make a profit (*fangquan rangli*).[11] For instance, through the *Notice of Strengthening the Economic Management of Hospitals*[12] (issued in 1979 and updated in 1981), economic incentive strategies were applied to produce motivations for work. In some hospitals, departments like dentistry, dermatology, and reproductive health were shifted to a contract responsibility system, with medical workers' income linked to output. Hospitals were even allowed make profits from drugs and high technology equipments and treatments (Liu et al., 2006). These new measures, recognized by then-Minister of Health Cui Yueli (崔月犁) and later diffused across provinces in China,[13] helped ease the state's financial burden, but market logic gradually impeded the management of the public hospitals in China.

On the demand side, removing the referral system allowed patients to pour directly into high-level hospitals equipped with more expensive technologies and

---

[10] See, for instance, A review of the economic and social development achievements of the 60th anniversary of the founding of New China, https://www.gov.cn/gzdt/2009-09/07/content_1410926.htm, accessed on September 15, 2023.

[11] See, for instance, the Decision of the Central Committee of the Communist Party of China on Economic System Reform issued on 1984, https://www.gov.cn/test/2008-06/26/content_1028140.htm, accessed on September 12, 2023.

[12] See, for instance, Notice on strengthening the pilot work of hospital economic management issued in 1979, http://www.reformdata.org/1979/0428/5223.shtml, accessed on September 12, 2023.

[13] See, for instance, History back and forth: public hospital reform from 1978 to 1992, http://m.chinareform.net/index.php?m=content&c=index&a=show&catid=59&id=39159, accessed on September 12, 2023.

sophisticated healthcare professionals (e.g., See Liu & Hsiao, 1995). China lost its well-functioning referral system in the transition period and became a client-based choice system (Eggleston et al., 2008). According to Yao (2016), under the planned economy, citizens needed to visit a community-based health service station first to receive a treatment referral; under the market model, one could go directly to a higher-level hospital for medical treatment without barriers, worsening the inequality in the distribution of health resources. As a consequence, higher-tier hospitals received more financial subsidies, higher talented personnel quotas, and more advanced health equipment and were usually located in large cities. China had transitioned to a market-oriented health system.

At the same time, the over-emphasis on economic returns reshaped healthcare professionals' behaviors. The shrinking government subsidies introduced commercial logic and motivated healthcare professionals to engage in for-profit behaviors, at odds with their non-profit nature. Hence, scandals like red pockets (patient bribing doctors as informal payment), kickbacks, extra bonuses, and medical disputes have been increasingly reported in the media since the 1990s (Bloom et al., 2001). Since the 2000s, a saying has spread by word-of-mouth among the public: "It is hard to see a doctor; it is expensive to see the doctor (*kanbingnan, kanbinggui* 看病难, 看病贵)".

The changes also exposed China's insufficient health insurance coverage system. In rural areas, removing the people's commune[14] led to the swift decline of the cooperative medical scheme (CMS), from 92.8% coverage in 1976 to 52.8% in 1982 (Wang, 2009). In some regions, the CMS was considered a "legacy" of 1960s leftist ideology; in others, local governments could no longer afford the health cost due to the breakdown of the rural collective economy. This left many rural residents devoid of mutual-help health insurance. Additionally, due to their increased financial autonomy and market competition, many state-owned enterprises (SOEs) experienced difficulties or went bankrupt, leading to a decline in laborers' health insurance coverage. The health insurance coverage rate fell from 32.3% in 1991 to 21.9% in 2000 (Li, Malik and Hu, 2017). The marketized health system and insufficient health insurance coverage worsened the health system in China. Facing public demands to maintain health services in the new century and bottom-up grievances, health reform in China became an urgent concern.

In 2009, Chinese authorities launched a new health reform program. To revitalize the for-publicness of public hospitals, the government initially limited medicine markups in hospitals to 15% in 2006 before banning them in 2017.[15] Meanwhile, to ease the workload of health professionals in higher-level hospitals and improve the health system at grassroots, the government also re-introduced primary health services at the community level, promoting the referral system. More importantly,

[14] In 1958, people's commune was estalibshed in rural China as a new political and economic organization, to realize the goal of complete state ownership of farms and mobilize the villagers.

[15] See, for instance, Completely cancel drug markups, the medical reform has sounded the clarion call, https://www.gov.cn/xinwen/2017-12/28/content_5251288.htm, accessed on September 12, 2023.

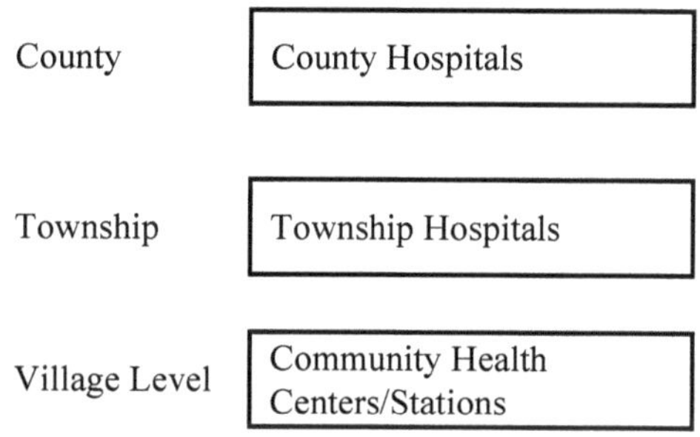

Fig. 1.2 Three-tier Health Delivery Services in Rural China. *Source* Summarized based on Chen Zhu (2009), Lancet

according to then-Minister of Health Chen Zhu (2009), the Chinese authority aimed to provide universal medical insurance coverage to 90% of the Chinese population, including urban residents, migrant workers, and peasants. The reformed universal health insurance coverage comprised three schemes. First, a new Rural Cooperative Medical Scheme (NRCMS) was introduced to provide health insurance to the rural population and address the vast inequalities between rural and urban residents. With increased central and local government subsidies, coverage increased from less than 10% in 2003 to 98.9% in 2013. Meanwhile, in urban settings, urban residence insurance continued to function. Third, employee-based health insurance was co-funded by employers and employees in both private and public sectors, reflecting pluralism in welfare provision (Fig. 1.2).

However, though significant improvements in the health system have been achieved, challenges remain. According to the 2021 Statistical Bulletin of China's Health System, the hospital bed occupancy rate of third-tier hospitals increased from 81.3% to 85.3%, compared to the 71.1% in second-tier hospitals and 52.1% in first-tier hospitals which also remained stagnant.[16] The goal of the three-tier health system aimed to increase the efficient utilization of primary health facilities, while the reality was contrary to the design. Citizens' health-seeking behaviors remain unchanged, and primary health institutions are still in low use. The reasons are two folded. Subjectively, although community health centers were designed to refer patients to higher-level hospitals when necessary, thousands of citizens still directly seek help from higher-level hospitals in big cities (Zhang et al., 2011). The perceived service quality gap between second- and third-tier hospitals remained (Shi et al., 2021). Attracted by superstitions about and trust in top-ranking hospitals reinforced the patients' health-seeking behaviors. Meanwhile, objectively, due to China's imbalanced health resource distribution (Zhao et al., 2020), there remained unequal spatial accessibility to hospitals between rural and urban, as well as between capital cities and the rest. Healthcare professionals in primary health institutions received inadequate training and qualifications, lower wages, and fewer appliances of advanced equipment (Li et al., 2017), which also dampened the development of the primary health system. Rural and non-local residents often seek medical help and second

[16] See, for instance, Statistical Communiqué on the Development of China's Health Care Industry in 2021, https://www.gov.cn/xinwen/2022-07/12/content_5700670.htm, accessed on October 4, 2023.

opinions from tertiary hospitals in larger cities, leaving them packed with patients daily.[17] As a consequence, in megacities, such as Beijing, Shanghai, Guangzhou, Wuhan, etc., the third-tier health institutions have been overloaded.

In addition, trust in healthcare professionals is diminishing due to repeated media reports of medical scandals. For instance, in 2015, Chinese authorities accused a famous U.K. pharmaceutical company, GSK, of using the travel agency network to bribe hospital health workers.[18] The company organized a medical conference, offering health workers monetary incentives and luxury treatment to give talks or receive training; in return, the health workers would boost the sales volume of GSK prescription products. As Tam Waikeung (2012) revealed, media exposure is correlated to distrust in professionals, with suspicions surrounding the relations between pharmaceutical companies and health workers and the high price of imported drugs arousing patients' dissatisfaction. Overall, the "people's doctors" (*renmin de yisheng* 人民的医生) have become a thing of the past; healthcare professionals have shifted from serving the people to serving the market (Yang, 2010). Public hospitals, while still public organs, now function more like self-sufficient enterprises.

When high expectations towards hospitals meet overworked healthcare professionals, the resulting unsatisfactory healthcare outcomes disappoint and frustrate patients. Sometimes, patients even turn their grievances into violence, leading to medical disturbances in public hospitals. These healthcare professionals sometimes become "scapegoats" for the inefficient and imperfect health system. What explains the occurrence of hospital violence in public hospitals? In the subsequent chapters, I use the case of hospital violence in the workplace to explain the political and social roots of social disturbances in public hospitals. In addition, I examine the interactions between patients, doctors, and local government and their informal agents. Constrained by their identification with public institutions and lack of organizational skills, doctors often faced strong pressure from the government and patients to remain "silent", meaning we rarely hear much from health workers. This book observes and investigates the various strategies, mindsets, and actions among the government, health professionals, and patients to reveal the overall picture of the medical disputes and social environment in China.

1.4 Methods

The study of popular resistance in China largely employs the single-case approach. Through the process-tracing approach, scholars show the contentious image of contemporary China. However, few examine the pattern of dispute resolution

---

[17] See, for instance, China's Health Care Crisis: Lines Before Dawn, Violence and 'No Trust', https://www.nytimes.com/2018/09/30/business/china-health-care-doctors.html, accessed on September 13, 2023.

[18] See, for instance, Four GlaxoSmithKline executives arrested, one suspected of accepting sexual bribes, http://politics.people.com.cn/n/2013/0715/c1001-22196936.html, accessed on September 13, 2023.

outcomes and systematically investigate the efficacy of disputants' strategies because of data availability. Hence, this book adopts a mixed-method approach involving over 700 archival cases that went through authorized non-legal mediation channels, 155 hospital violence cases and their legal outcomes, and 72 in-depth interviews obtained through fieldwork in Megacity C in China from 2015 to 2017.

Qualitatively, I conducted in-depth interviews with various stakeholders, including doctors, nurses, patients, police officers, and hospital security guards. Interviewees were front-line workers who routinely dealt with disputes; however, their voices are missing from extant studies. I also spoke to district- and municipal-level juridical system representatives to discuss the future of the medical dispute resolution process. All interviews were semi-structured and lasted at least 30 min, subject to the subject's availability.

Quantitatively, I collected cases of hospital violence from across China and traced the punishment received from the juridical system. I observed the daily practice of justice and government interventions towards hospital violence as a law-breaking behavior in China. Using a keyword search, I collected published reports of 155 incidents of hospital violence in the workplace from 2010 to 2017 from the China Digital Library database and other mainstream newspapers. Detailed information was captured for each instance, including the nature of the violence they applied, the duration of the hospital violence, the patient's tactics, and its outcome (government responses) to empirically trace the legal outcomes of citizens' law-breaking behaviors. I also examined government officials' diversified strategies and complex mindsets in dealing with hospital violence (See Appendix).

Indeed, extreme cases, such as hospital violence, rarely happen. In addition to examining extreme hospital violence against doctors, I analyze regular medical disputes and associated institutional responses. With the help of local collaborators, I contacted local justice departments and, with their cooperation, carried out fieldwork in the mediation dispute mediation committee, a new institution carrying Maoist justice genes designed to resolve medical disputes through an extra-legal approach, also known as the legacy of "People's Mediation". The committees are the authorized channel for dealing with disputes between patients and hospitals through which I compiled mediation case-level data. The detailed archival case data allowed me to study variances in patients' compensation outcomes and helped me observe institutional responses towards medical disputes in their daily practices. The first-hand data and valuable archival documents help depict citizens' social dispute resolution process in China.

During the summer and winter months from 2015 to 2017, I conducted ethnographic fieldwork in a metropolitical city in China equipped with the best health and legal resources for citizens. As most health resources are more plentiful in urban areas, so are the chances of medical disputes occurring. The city was chosen as the setting for this research for two reasons. First, it is one of the first regions to experiment with using mediation channel for medical dispute resolution. Since 2011, the C government has pioneered using specialized mediation services to intervene in the medical dispute resolution process. Second, the region is known for its high mediation rate and efficiency; patients often agree to accept reduced compensation after

Table 1.2 Mediate success rate from 2013 to 2017 in the city C

	2013		2014		2015		2016		2017	
	No	%	No	%	No	%	No	%	No	%
Mediated Cases	132	83	141	91	132	85	145	86	112	93
Litigation	6	4	5	3	6	4	0	0	0	0
Others	20	13	9	6	17	11	23	14	8	7
Total	158	100	155	100	155	100	68	100	120	100

Note Success rate, in this book, refers to dispute cases in which a legally binding agreement is reached

mediation, and none of the cases that went through mediation have led to further collective actions. The region's overall mediation success rate rose from 83% in 2012 to 93% in 2016, higher than the national average. Therefore, C region was a suitable backdrop for examining mediators' dynamic strategies and the efficacy of mediation institutions (Table 1.2).

1.5 Overview of the Book

This study aims to explain and examine the dynamic government-citizen relationship in the transition era—in particular, why and how social disputes evolved into confrontations between citizens and government in contemporary China. Social disputes have the potential to evolve into collective actions with heightened emotion from citizens, and disputants with grievances often refashion their target from public institutions or private enterprises to the government to redress their grievances or support their claims. To decipher what turns medical disputes between patients and doctors into social conflicts between citizens and authorities, I begin with a history of dispute resolution institutions in China. Many medical disputes often contain disruptive behaviors, also known as non-compliance behaviors. Hence, in this study, hospital violence is considered an extreme form of medical dispute, often involving individual or collective violence and law-breaking activities.

Chapter 2 reviews the politicization process of medical dispute resolution in China since the reform and opening up. It also provides a history of mediation committees from an institutional change perspective. Looking into the social dispute resolution process may reveal the changing attitudes and strategies the government has applied to manage social disputes. The preference for mediation channels over legal ones dates back to the revolutionary era. In 1940, especially in the border region of Shaan-Gan-Ning (陕甘宁边区), where Mao decided the model of a new China was to be built, the trend of "Ma Xiwu's way of Judging" (马锡五判案) emerged and was praised. Ma Xiwu's way refers to combining mediation and litigation as an alternative to local courts (Cong, 2014). The process allowed vanguard cadres to replace the social gentry and affluent families and build a micropower base in everyday politics.

This tradition prevailed in the Mao era since mediation institutions coincided with the crystallization of the mass line. In the post-Mao era, legal institutions were revived. Although legal institutions, with restricted reform, are still regarded as a functional department of the Party-state to exercise social control (Liebman, 2017), their reappearance has unexpectedly advanced citizens' legal consciousness and willingness to adopt legal measures in dispute resolution, leading to the fall of mediation institutions. However, we have now witnessed the return of mediation, combined with the mass line strategy and rule-of-law rhetoric. By tracing the historical rise and fall of the mediation channel, this chapter allows us to comb the changing attitudes of the Party-state towards the rule of law and dispute resolution in China.

Chapters 3–5 provide the intensive ethnographic details of medical dispute resolution and the power embedded when social dispute resolution was politicized. Chapter 3 examines extreme medical disputes—hospital violence—in China and summarizes the strategies of hospital violence and the political space that enables non-compliance behaviors in China. It theoretically analyzes hospital violence from the political participation perspective, which provides a new lens to extant studies mainly centered on the medical field. Through case study, this chapter examines how fragmented local-level law enforcement, local officials' moral duty, and patients' strategic choices have shaped the heterogeneous consequences of non-compliance behaviors. It advances our understanding of inconsistent law enforcement at street level.

Chapter 4 examines strategic and non-coercive government responses to medical disputes in China by investigating the strategies of mediators as informal government agents. Instead of resorting to repression, as widely discussed in the extant scholarship, the socialist regime has invented a series of institutionalized channels—mediation committees—to address social disputes. This book examines the art of persuasion by observing the mediators' strategies in medical dispute resolution. Through participatory observation, it discloses the dispute resolution process and how mediators utilize their multiple identities as friends, semi-officials, and legal experts as affective, political, and legal strategies to facilitate the dispute mediation process. It advances our understanding of how mediation prevails in China and is preferred by the government to solve social disputes without resorting to coercion and direct government intervention.

Chapter 5 examines how the government has applied monetary compensation to shift the focus of medical disputes from rights protection to economic bargaining and the efficacy thereof by reviewing dispute cases. Little systematic evidence exists to explain the government's compensation distribution rationale or strategic objectives in pursuing compensation distribution to settle social disputes, especially those between citizens and the government or its agents. This book investigates the compensation distribution rationale using the unique dataset collected from the fieldwork and unveils the process of "buying stability." The author finds that the mediation committees played the role of a centralized bargaining channel and that monetary distribution outcomes were shaped by distributive justice, political stability pressure, and economic cost concerns.

Chapter 6 reflects on the implications and theoretical contributions of politicized social dispute resolution and advances our understanding of changing state-society relations in contemporary China. Specifically, it advances our understanding of China's politicized social dispute resolution institutions and processes and examines the government's strategic responses to disruptive actions. Since the government needed to maintain social stability and show mercy to the people with grievances, it largely refrained from using coercive repression. However, the creation, process, and outcome of social dispute resolutions are all shaped by political factors. The government must constantly balance the often contradictory demands of the rule of law, morality, and political stability.

This study brings the cultural perspective back to the center of the study of contentious politics. It contributes to understanding the newly articulated new state-society relations by disclosing daily government-citizen interactions. Through the frequent use of the buying stability strategy, personal interest-based petitioning and government monetary compensation have commercialized state-society relations and could, in the long run, breed regime instability rather than contribute to regime stability as expected.

This study also joins discussions of the rule of law in China. As Minzner (2011) said, Chinese authorities are "turning against the law" by preferring mediation over trials according to the law (p. 943). I agree that the Maoist tradition of mediation has diluted the principle of the rule of law, but I also find that the new institutionalized mediation channel combines the mass-line tradition with professional features to balance politics and the rule of law. This book suggests that informal and non-legal institutions (such as social institutions) have played a crucial and necessary role in facilitating dispute resolution efficiently in China. It provides evidence on how the informal institutions have shaped selective law enforcement at the street level. It dives into the debate of the perception of justice among Chinese citizens in dispute resolution, which largely relied on the personal efficacy in the legal system. It sheds light on how mediation institutions contribute not only to dispute resolution but the resilience as well. The chapter concludes with projections about the future of doctor-patient relations and the landscape of social dispute resolution.

References

Benney, J. (2016) Weiwen at the Grassroots: China's stability maintenance apparatus as a means of conflict resolution. *Journal of Contemporary China, 25*(99): 389–405.

Blecher, M. J. (2002) Hegemony and workers' politics in China. *The China Quarterly*, 170: 283–303.

Bloom, G., Han, L., & Li, X. (2001) How health workers earn a living in China. *Human Resources for Health Development Journal*, *5*(1-3): 25–38. https://opendocs.ids.ac.uk/opendocs/bitstream/handle/20.500.12413/3439/Wp108.pdf?sequence=1.

Cai, Y. (2002) The resistance of Chinese laid-off workers in the reform period. *The China Quarterly, 170*(2): 327–344.

Cai, Y. (2005) China's moderate middle class: the case of homeowners' resistance. *Asian Survey, 45*(5): 777–799.

Cai, Y. (2008) Power structure and regime resilience: contentious politics in China. *British Journal of Political Science*, *38*(3): 411–432.
Cai, Y. (2020) *Collective resistance in China: Why popular protests succeed or fail.* Stanford University Press.
Chan, C. S. C. (2018) Mistrust of physicians in China: society, institution, and interaction as root causes. *Developing world bioethics 18*(1): 16–25.
Chan, C. S.-c., & Yao, Z. (2018) A market of distrust: toward a cultural sociology of unofficial exchanges between patients and doctors in China. Theory and Society, 47(6): 737–772.
Chen, B. (2004) "Chansu, xinfang yu xinzhongguo falv chuantong falv chuangxingqi de chansu wenti" ("Persistant Lawsuits, Xinfang, and Legal tradition in PRC: The issues of persistant lawsuits in the period of legal transformation"). *Peking University Law Journal*, *16*(2): 226–238.
Chen, F. (2003) Between the state and labour: The conflict of Chinese trade unions' double identity in market reform. The China Quarterly, 176: 1006–1028.
Chen, M. S. (2001) The great reversal: transformation of health care in the People's Republic of China, in The Blackwell companion to medical sociology. William C. Cockerham, Blackwell Publishers, 456–482.
Chen, X. (2009) The power of "troublemaking": protest tactics and their efficacy in China. *Comparative Politics*, *41*(4): 451–471.
Chen, X. (2012) *Social protest and contentious authoritarianism in China.* Cambridge University Press.
Chen, X. (2020) Civic and Noncivic Activism under Autocracy: Shifting Political Space for Popular Collective Action. *Mobilization: An International Quarterly*, *25*(SI): 623–640.
Chen, Z. (2009) Launch of the health-care reform plan in China. *The Lancet*, *373*(9672), 1322–1324.
Cong, X. (2014) "Ma Xiwu's Way of Judging": Villages, the Masses and Legal Construction in Revolutionary China in the 1940s. *The China Journal*(72): 29–52.
Davenport, C. (2005) Understanding covert repressive action: The case of the US government against the Republic of New Africa. *Journal of Conflict Resolution*, *49*(1), 120–140.
Davis, D. S. (2000) Social class transformation in urban China: training, hiring, and promoting urban professionals and managers after 1949. Modern China, 26(3): 251–275
Diamant, N. J., & O'Brien, K. J. (2015) Veterans' political activism in China. *Modern China, 41*(3): 278–312.
Dimitrov, M. (2008) The resilient authoritarians. *Current History*, *107*(705): 24–29.
Distelhorst, G. (2017) The power of empty promises: Quasi-democratic institutions and activism in China. *Comparative Political Studies, 50*(4): 464–498.
Earl, J. (2003) Tanks, tear gas, and taxes: Toward a theory of movement repression. *Sociological theory*, *21*(1): 44–68.
Earl, J. (2011) Political repression: Iron fists, velvet gloves, and diffuse control. *Annual review of sociology*, *37*: 261–284.
Eggleston, K., Ling, L., Qingyue, M., Lindelow, M., & Wagstaff, A. (2008) Health service delivery in China: a literature review. *Health economics, 17*(2): 149–165.
Fan Yu. (2000) "Fei susong jiufen jiejue jizhi yanjiu" *(Alternative dispute resolution mechanism research)* (China Renmin University Press).
Fang, Q. (2009) China's Current Mail and Visit System and Its Fundamental Predicament. *Modern China Studies*, *16*(4) https://www.modernchinastudies.org/cn/issues/past-issues/106-mcs-2009-issue-4/1113-chinas-current-mail-and-visit-system-and-its-fundamental-predicament.html.
Feng Shizheng. (2012) "Guojia zhengquan jianshe yu xinzhongguo xinfang zhidudexingcheng yu yanbian" ("State Building and the Installation and Change of the Xinfang System in China Since 1949") *(Sociological Studies)*, *4*: 25–47.
Field, M. G. (1991) The hybrid profession: Soviet medicine. In *Professions and the state: expertise and autonomy in the Soviet Union and Eastern Europe*, edited by MG Field, Jones A., Temple University Press: 43–62.
Freidson, E. (1984) The changing nature of professional control. *Annual review of sociology*, 1–20.

Fu, H. (2015) Between deference and defiance: courts and penal populism in Chinese capital cases. In *The Death Penalty in China: Policy, Practice, and Reform*, edited by Liang, B., & Lu, H., Columbia University Press, 274–299.

Fu, D., & Distelhorst, G. (2018) Grassroots participation and repression under Hu Jintao and Xi Jinping. The China Journal, 79(1): 100–122.

Gallagher, M. (2017) *Authoritarian legality in China: Law, workers, and the state*: Cambridge University Press.

Gallagher, M. E. (2006) Mobilizing the law in China:"Informed disenchantment" and the development of legal consciousness. *Law & Society Review*, *40*(4): 783–816.

Gao, X. (2012) Between the state and the private sphere: Chinese state medicine movement, 1930–1949. In *Science, public health and the state in modern Asia, edited by Bu, L., Stapleton, D. H., & Yip, K. C.*, Taylor & Francis, 144–160.

He, A. J. (2014) The doctor–patient relationship, defensive medicine and overprescription in Chinese public hospitals: Evidence from a cross-sectional survey in Shenzhen city. *Social science & medicine, 123*: 64–71.

He, A. J., & Qian, J. (2016) Explaining medical disputes in Chinese public hospitals: the doctor–patient relationship and its implications for health policy reforms. *Health Economics, Policy and Law, 11*(4): 359–378.

Henderson, G., & Cohen, M. S. (1984) The Chinese hospital: A socialist work unit. (New Haven: Yale University Press).

Hobsbawm, E. J. (1974) Social banditry. In *Rural protest: peasant movements and social change* (pp. 142–157) London: Palgrave Macmillan UK.

Hsiao, W. C. (1995) The Chinese health care system: lessons for other nations. *Social science & medicine, 41*(8): 1047–1055.

Hu, J. (2011) Grand mediation in China. *Asian Survey, 51*(6): 1065–1089.

Huang, H., Boranbay-Akan, S., & Huang, L. (2019) Media, protest diffusion, and authoritarian resilience. *Political Science Research and Methods, 7*(1): 23–42.

Huang, P. C. (1993) " Public Sphere"/" Civil Society" in China? The Third Realm between State and Society. *Modern China, 19*(2): 216–240.

Hurst, W., Liu, M., Liu, Y., & Tao, R. (2014) Reassessing collective petitioning in rural China: civic engagement, extra-state violence, and regional variation. *Comparative politics, 46*(4): 459–482.

Koss, D. (2021) Party building as institutional bricolage: asserting authority at the business frontier. *The China Quarterly, 248*(S1): 222–243.

Kuang, X., & Göbel, C. (2013) Sustaining collective action in urbanizing China. *The China Quarterly, 216*: 850–871.

Kumar, M., Verma, M., Das, T., Pardeshi, G., Kishore, J., & Padmanandan, A. (2016) A study of workplace violence experienced by doctors and associated risk factors in a tertiary care hospital of South Delhi, India. *Journal of clinical and diagnostic research: JCDR, 10*(11), LC06.

Lampton, D. M. (1977) The politics of medicine in China: the policy process 1949–1977, Westview Press.

Lee, C. K. (2007) *Against the law: Labor protests in China's rustbelt and sunbelt*: Univ of California Press.

Lee, C. K., & Zhang, Y. (2013) The power of instability: Unraveling the microfoundations of bargained authoritarianism in China. *American journal of sociology, 118*(6): 1475–1508.

Lei, Y. W., & Zhou, D. X. (2015) Contesting legality in authoritarian contexts: food safety, rule of law and China's networked public sphere. *Law & Society Review, 49*(3): 557–593.

Leung, J. C., & Nann, R. C. (1995) *Authority and benevolence: Social welfare in China.* Chinese University Press.

Li, L. (2006) Driven to protest: China's rural unrest. *Current History, 105*(692): 250–254.

Li, L. (2010) Rights consciousness and rules consciousness in contemporary China. *The China Journal*, (64): 47–68.

Li, L., Liu, M., & O'Brien, K. J. (2012) Petitioning Beijing: the high tide of 2003–2006. *The China Quarterly, 210*, 313–334.

Li, Y., Malik, V., & Hu, F. B. (2017) Health insurance in China: after declining in the 1990s, coverage rates rebounded to near-universal levels by 2011. *Health Affairs, 36*(8): 1452–1460.

Li, X., Lu, J., Hu, S., Cheng, K. K., De Maeseneer, J., Meng, Q., ... & Hu, S. (2017) The primary health-care system in China. *The Lancet, 390*(10112): 2584–2594.

Liebman, B. L. (2007) China's Courts: Restricted Reform, 21 Colum. *J. Asian L, 1*. Available at: https://scholarship.law.columbia.edu/faculty_scholarship/3374.

Liebman, B. L. (2013) Malpractice mobs: medical dispute resolution in China. *Columbia Law Review*: 181–264.

Liebman, B. L. (2015) Leniency in Chinese Criminal Law: Everyday Justice in Henan. *Berkeley J. Int'l L., 33*, 153, Available at: https://scholarship.law.columbia.edu/faculty_scholarship/1085.

Liebman, B. L. (2017) China's courts: Restricted reform. In *Law and society in East Asia* (pp. 237–280) Routledge.

Liu, X., & Hsiao, W. C. (1995) The cost escalation of social health insurance plans in China: its implication for public policy. *Social science & medicine, 41*(8): 1095–1101.

Liu, Y., Berman, P., Yip, W., Liang, H., Meng, Q., Qu, J., & Li, Z. (2006) Health care in China: the role of non-government providers. Health Policy, 77(2): 212–220.

Lorentzen, P. (2017) Designing contentious politics in post-1989 China. *Modern China, 43*(5): 459–493.

Lorentzen, P. L. (2013) Regularizing rioting: Permitting public protest in an authoritarian regime. *Quarterly Journal of Political Science, 8*(2): 127–158.

Luo, Q., & Andreas, J. (2016) Using Religion to Resist Rural Dispossession: A Case Study of a Hui Muslim Community in North-west China. *The China Quarterly, 226*: 477–498.

Meng, T., Pan, J., & Yang, P. (2017) Conditional receptivity to citizen participation: Evidence from a survey experiment in China. Comparative Political Studies, 50(4): 399–433.

Minzner, C. F. (2006) Xinfang: an alternative to formal Chinese legal institutions. *Stan. J. Int'l l., 42*, 103. Available at: http://ir.lawnet.fordham.edu/faculty_scholarship/3

Ng, K. H., & He, X. (2017) *Embedded courts: Judicial decision-making in China*. Cambridge University Press.

Minzner, C. F. (2011) China's turn against law. *The American Journal of Comparative Law, 59*(4): 935–984.

O'brien, K. J. (1996) Rightful resistance. *World Politics, 49*(1): 31–55.

O'Brien, K. J. (2002) Collective action in the Chinese countryside. The China Journal 48: 139–154.

O'Brien, K. J. (2013) Rightful resistance revisited. *Journal of Peasant Studies, 40*(6): 1051–1062.

O'brien, K. J., & Li, L. (2000) Accommodating "democracy" in a one-party state: Introducing village elections in China. *The China Quarterly, 162*: 465–489.

O'Brien, K. J., & Li, L. (2006) *Rightful resistance in rural China*: Cambridge University Press.

Pan, P. (2002) In China, turning the law into the people's protector. *The Washington Post, 28*, A01.

Pengyu Zhao et al. (2018) "Menzhen huanzhe dui yihuanguanxi d renzhi xianzhuang ji yingxiang yinsu fenxi" ("Analysis of the current cognitive status of outpatients on the doctor-patient relationship and its influencing factors"). (Chinese Hospital Management Journal), 34 (2): 123–127. https://doi.org/10.3760/cma.j.issn.1000-6672.2018.02.008.

Pepinsky, T. B. (2013) Pluralism and political conflict in Indonesia. *Indonesia*, (96), 81–100.

Pepinsky, T. (2014) The institutional turn in comparative authoritarianism. *British Journal of Political Science, 44*(3): 631–653.

Perry, E. J. (2008) Chinese conceptions of "rights": From Mencius to Mao—and now. *Perspectives on Politics, 6*(1): 37–50.

Perry, E. J. (2009) A new rights consciousness?. *J. Democracy, 20*, 17.

Perry, E. J. (2012) Anyuan: mining China's revolutionary tradition (Vol. 24) Univ of California Press.

Perry, E. J., & Selden, M. (2000) Reform and resistance in contemporary China. *Chinese society, change, conflict and resistance, 2*.

Schram, S., & Chinnery, J. (1974) *Chairman Mao talks to the people: talks and letters 1956–1971*: Pantheon Books. A division of Random House.

Scott, J. C. (1985) *Weapons of the weak: Everyday forms of peasant resistance.* yale university Press.
Shi, H., Fan, M., Zhang, H., Ma, S., Wang, W., Yan, Z., & Bi, R. (2021) Perceived health-care quality in China: a comparison of second-and third-tier hospitals. *International Journal for Quality in Health Care, 33*(1), mzab027.
Sidel, V. W. (1972) The barefoot doctors of the People's Republic of China. *New England Journal of Medicine, 286*(24): 1292–1300.
Sheng, Z. (2017) Organizational mobilization, action strategy and opportunity structure: Factors affecting the results of homeowners' collective actions. *Chinese journal of sociology, 3*(4): 548–580.
Shi, F., & Cai, Y. (2006) Disaggregating the state: networks and collective resistance in Shanghai. *The China Quarterly, 186*: 314–332.
Tam, W. (2012) Health care reform and patients' trust in physicians in urban Beijing. *The China Quarterly, 211*: 827–843.
Tsai, L. L. (2015) Constructive Noncompliance. *Comparative politics, 47*(3): 253–279.
Wagstaff, A., Yip, W., Lindelow, M., & Hsiao, W. C. (2009) China's health system and its reform: a review of recent studies. Health economics, 18(S2): S7–S23.
Wang, S. (2009) Adapting by learning: the evolution of China's rural health care financing. *Modern China, 35*(4): 370–404.
Wang, V. L. (1975) Training of the barefoot doctor in the People's Republic of China: from prevention to curative service. International Journal of Health Services, 5(3): 475–488.
Wang, Y., & Minzner, C. (2015) The rise of the Chinese security state. The China Quarterly, 222: 339–359.
Xu, W. (2014) Violence against doctors in China. The Lancet, 384(9945), 745.
Yang, J. (2010) Serve the people: understanding ideology and professional ethics of medicine in China. *Health Care Analysis, 18*(3): 294–309.
Yang, K. (2022) Mobilizing without Solidarity: Sustained Activism among Chinese Veterans. *The China Journal, 87*(1): 1–19.
Yang, K. (2023) Beyond parochial activism: cross-regional protests and the changing landscape of popular contention in China. *Journal of Contemporary China, 32*(140), 280–295.
Yao Zelin. (2015) "Jindai yilai zhongguo yisheng zhiye yu guojia guanxi de yanbian —yizhong zhiye shehuixue de jieshi" ("The Changing Relationship between Chinese Urban Medical Profession and the State since the republican Period: From the perspective of the sociology of professions") (*Sociological Studies*), (3): 46–68.
Yao Zelin (2016) "Xingzheng, shichang yu zhiye: chengshi fenji zhenliao de sanzhongzhilimoshi jiqi shijian" ("The evolution of the relationship between the Chinese medical profession and the state in modern times—an explanation from professional sociology") (Social Science), 6: 84–93.
Yip, W. C.-M., Hsiao, W., Meng, Q., Chen, W., & Sun, X. (2010) Realignment of incentives for health-care providers in China. *The Lancet, 375*(9720): 1120–1130.
Yu, J. (2005) "xinfang zhidu gaige yu xianzheng jianshe" ("Reform of the petition system and construction of constitutional government") *(Twenty-First Century), 6.*
Yu, J. (2016) "wo weishenm zhuzhang feichu xinfang zhidu" (Why do I advocate the abolition of Xinfang system?) See, http://www.aisixiang.com/data/99255.html.
Zelizer, V. A. (2018) Human values and the market: The case of life insurance and death in 19th-century America. In *The sociology of economic life* (pp. 125–140) Routledge.
Zelizer, V. A. R. (2017) *Morals and markets: The development of life insurance in the United States.* Columbia University Press.
Zhang, Y. M. (1999) China health course for 50 years. Beijing: the Public House of Ancient Works. cited in Wang, J. H. (2015). Medical System Reforms in China after 1978: Some Practical Implications. In *2nd Annual International Conference on Social Science and Contemporary Humanity Development* (pp. 646–654) Atlantis Press.

Zhang, J., & Cai, Y. (2019) Medical disputes and mediation in China: Government and responsibility shifting. *China Information, 33*(3): 350–371.
Zhang, X., Chen, L. W., Mueller, K., Yu, Q., Liu, J., & Lin, G. (2011) Tracking the effectiveness of health care reform in China: a case study of community health centers in a district of Beijing. *Health Policy, 100*(2–3): 181–188.
Zedong Mao 1996. "Mao Zedong Wenji" (Collected works of Mao Zedong) Volume 3. (Renmin Press).
Zhong, Y., & Hwang, W. (2016) Pollution, Institutions and Street Protests in Urban China. *Journal of Contemporary China, 25*(98): 216–232.
Zhou, X. (2017) From China's "Barefoot Doctor" to Alma Ata: The Primary Health Care Movement in the Long 1970s. *China, Hong Kong, and the long 1970s: Global perspectives*, 135–157.
Zhou, X. (2020) *The People's Health: Health Intervention and Delivery in Mao's China 1949–1983* (Vol. 2) McGill-Queen's Press-MQUP.
Zhao, P., Li, S., & Liu, D. (2020) Unequable spatial accessibility to hospitals in developing megacities: New evidence from Beijing. *Health & Place, 65*, 102406.
Zhuang, W., & Chen, F. (2015) "Mediate First": The revival of mediation in labour dispute resolution in China. *The China Quarterly, 222*: 380–402.

Chapter 2
Politicized Medical Dispute Resolution

How did medical dispute resolution become politicized in China? This chapter examines the changing landscape of medical dispute resolution from the 1990s to Xi's current reign. It documents the changing strategies and attitudes the government applied and adaptative institutions in absorbing and managing social disputes in China. In the 1990s, bureaucratic concerns and the underdeveloped legal system constrained citizens' agency in holding hospitals and doctors accountable. Since 2002, under the rule of law, the new Medical Malpractice Regulation has encouraged patients to use the law as a weapon to address their disputes. However, legal channels are a double-edged sword. Law mobilization has coincided with the high tide of rights protection, leading to increased dispute cases against hospitals, and even collective actions targeting public health institutions. The fragmented responses to social disputes fail to address the citizens' grievance and yet further destabilize the regime. Today, to maintain social stability, social dispute resolution institutions have been institutionalized, adapted from legal channels to a traditional Maoist weapon—People's Mediation Institutions. This chapter theorizes the mediation channel's institutional constraints and politicized outcomes. It explains how the dynamic interaction between the rule of law, social power, and stability maintenance influences the mediation channel in China.

J. Wu, *Politicized Medical Dispute Resolution in China*, Understanding China,
https://doi.org/10.1007/978-981-97-6961-2_2

2.1 Medical Dispute Resolution in the 1990s: Throw an Egg to the Stone

Medical dispute resolution has never been easy in China. After the reform and opening up, the State Council issued the *Medical Malpractice Regulation* in 1987[1] to regulate health institutions and empower citizens to dispute medical malpractice cases. However, suing doctors for medical malpractice was very difficult and rarely done. The definition of medical malpractice was narrow, resting on "whether healthcare professionals' negligence had *directly* caused the death, disability, and dysfunction of the patient" and ruling out medical negligence that led to less severe outcomes. The regulation placed the burden of proof on patients to limit or deter cases (Wang, 1999). As the criteria were highly specialized and difficult for laymen to navigate, courts primarily relied on technical medical examination reports from professional health institutions to decide and assign responsibility. Due to the interconnection between public hospitals and the health system (all public hospitals are sponsored by local governments and supervised by local health departments), it was like allowing a father to judge their son's behaviors. Even if medical malpractice was found, the disputant only received a one-time settlement fee and was not entitled to request compensation. In most regions, the one-time settlement fee ranged between 3000 and 6000 RMB,[2] not comparable to the loss of life. Public institutions' interests were often prioritized over those of patients.

The pattern of favoring hospitals was reinforced when the government downsized its financial support for the health system in the 1990s to encourage a free market system (Hsiao, 1995). With the retrenchment of government resources, Chinese healthcare has faced increasing financial challenges (Eggleston et al., 2008), and public hospitals have changed from state-owned work units to company-like enterprises. Some public hospitals have to invest in for-profit behaviors, including overtreatment, increased use of new equipment, and outsourcing to make ends meet and pay health workers (Hsiao, 1995). Healthcare professionals' iron bowls have been broken. The for-profit behaviors of healthcare professionals have also diluted the public nature of hospitals and reduced the quality of health services. To allow the health system to operate and survive, the government closed its eyes and effectively encouraged for-profit behaviors.

Meanwhile, healthcare professionals are wildly uneven in quality due to unequal healthcare reforms and financial resources (Lam et al., 2006). Some, especially those in underdeveloped regions or who received medical training during the Cultural Revolution, have not received sufficient and systematic medical training, often leading to misdiagnoses. Economic incentives and low quality of health services gave rise to frequent medical disputes. For instance, In an internal report, local officials in

---

[1] See, for instance, Regulation on medical malpractice, http://www.nhc.gov.cn/yzygj/s3576/200804/f62b22b1047f4f699c90733b8012a4ff.shtml, accessed on September 15, 2023.

[2] See for instance, The substantial increase in compensation standards in the new medical malpractice regulations has attracted the attention of all parties, https://fzggw.cq.gov.cn/zwxx/bmdt/202002/t20200212_5201205_wap.html, accessed on September 15, 2023.

Jiangsu's health department analyzed the causes of medical malpractice, drawing on fifteen local dispute cases, and found that the commercialization of health services hindered quality management in health institutions, especially in grassroots community health centers with limited resources (*weisheng yuan* 卫生院). The report commented that

> some work units focused on quantity of health service, rather than the quality; prioritized the hard goals of economic gains, instead of soft goals of quality. Some health workers have weak sense of responsibility. A few medical workers had not received systematic training and with lower professional level, which led to seven cases of misdiagnosis and wrong diagnosis (Chen & Yang, 1993, p.13).

Getting a medical malpractice case accepted is like "an ant trying to shake a tree" and long delays in local court often occur. For example, in Ningxia, on 18 July, 1995, Huang Liang (黄靓), the 18-year-old daughter of Huang Dejin (黄德金), died during an appendectomy surgery due to negligence in anesthetization, only a few days before she could have been officially admitted to Chongqing University (Cai, 2000).[3] The hospital, a secondary hospital affiliated with the mining company where Huang worked, denied Huang's request for an autopsy and refused to accept responsibility for the malpractice and offer any form of apology. After repeated medical technical examinations, the local health bureau deemed the death an accident rather than medical malpractice.

Due to the inter-connectedness between hospitals and supervisory institutions, medical technical reports are often biased in favor local public hospitals. Patients need to show proof of malpractice and a causal link between the negligence and death to justify the case, which is often impossible for a layman (Xiaobei, 1998). Huang spent three years self-studying medical knowledge, including clinical surgery, anesthesiology, and health regulations to determine the cause of his daughter's death, resulting in a 300,000-word research report. His persistence touched the nerves of many readers with the help of local media reports, earning him wide-spread sympathy and professional support from influential lawyers (e.g. Wu Jialin 吴家麟) and doctors (Tong, 2011). Though the legal process was prolonged and tiring, Huang was finally compensated after four years of persistent effort.

In fact, even when a case is accepted, local courts usually offer low compensation to protect the hospitals from economic loss or bankruptcy. In the 1987 *Medical Malpractice Regulation*, monetary compensation for malpractice was set at around 3000 RMB for first-level malpractice (causing death), varied by region. In developed areas, like Shanghai, compensation for citizens over 16 years old was no more than 4000 yuan, decreasing to less than 3000 yuan in Gansu province, a less developed region in Northwest China (Qiu, 1996). However, based on Article 119 of the *General Principles of Civil Law*,[4] issued the same year, citizens are entitled to receive

[3] See, for instance, Medical litigation is hard, https://www.gmw.cn/01shsb/1998-08/31/GB/723%5ESH14-309.htm, accessed on May 13, 2024.

[4] See, for instance, General Principles of Civil Law of the People's Republic of China, http://www.npc.gov.cn/zgrdw/npc/lfzt/rlys/2014-10/24/content_1882690.htm, accessed on September 15, 2023.

much higher compensation, possibly ten or a hundred times as much, exposing the underlying conflict between Civil Law and government promulgated regulations. In practice, courts often followed medical malpractice regulation standards to avoid placing a heavy financial burden or bankruptcy on hospitals. Putting a price on the human body is unacceptable in Chinese culture; setting the economic "value" of a human body at only 3000 RMB is even worse.

In 1989, in Urumqi, Liu Yin underwent an unnecessary fallopian tube surgery due to misdiagnosis (Yang, 2003). Due to this medical error, she was hospitalized for 42 days, costing her 3000 yuan. The local court asked the hospital to refund 3000 yaun, plus an additional 1000 yuan as one-time monetary compensation. Her appeal for another trial was dismissed. Similarly, in Tianjin 1984, a doctor mistakenly removed Li Xinrong's thyroid and parathyroid glands during surgery, making Li suffer from imbalanced hormones and reliant on lifelong medication treatment (Yang, 2003). Though the medical technical examination identified the case as a second-level medical technical error, the local court only gave a one-time payment of 5000 yuan as compensation, based on medical malpractice regulations. Luckily, the verdict was reversed in a second trial and Li received 570,000 yuan in compensation, based on the newly promogulated Civil Law.[5] However, that happened in August 1996, over a decade after the tragedy took place. From a legal perspective, a dual medical malpractice compensation system was in place, creating chaos and inconsistency in medical disputes (Wang & Oliphant, 2012). Sometimes, dualism even became the source of disputes, redirecting the patients' anger towards the courts and local governments.

When suing a doctor is difficult, citizens often shift their grievances to other channels as alternatives. Despite the nonprofit nature of health in China, the increasing user fees promoted citizens considering public health provision in China as a business and themselves as customers. Hence, from January 1996 to February 1997, the China Consumer Association (CCA) received 37 complaints about medical malpractice or disputes[6]; that number quadrupled in the following year's cycle. However, due to limited resources and capacity, the CCA could only pressure local government to intervene by exerting top-down administrative pressure such as sending an official letter and awaiting a possible reply. In 1997, the CCA sent 183 official letters to involved governments and hospitals, with only a 50% response rate.[7] The CCA channel's actual resolution rate was less than 6.5%.

Rapid economic reform and social change has changed China's health sector. Frequent reports of medical malpractice drew the Ministry of Health's attention, leading then-spokesman Zhi Junbo (支峻波) to declare a a media conference,

> Accompanied by the reform and open-up, the health industry has gone through development. However, too many reports were placed on medical disputes and the negative sides of the

[5] Later the hospital representative petitioned to the higher court, and finally ruled the hospital bear the medical expenses and compensation up to 250,000 yuan.

[6] See, for instance, Economic observation: Medical complaints become a hot topic, https://finance.sina.com.cn/management/vision/1999-9-9/5755.html, accessed on September 15, 2023.

[7] *Ibid.*

> reform. More media attention should shift to how the health sector adapted to the development needs of the socialist economy. Prior, we enjoyed free medical care as we rendered the health sector was considered as the welfare (non-profit) sector. Now, to accommodate to the changing society we need to raise the service charge of the medical care to boost the dynamic of health institutions to achieve both social and economic benefits.[8]

However, it failed to change the public's declining perception towards the quality of the health service provision in China. Meanwhile, the flood of medical disputes also exposed the limited institutional channels to address bottom-up grievances and discontent in the transition era. Courts were constrained to protect the interests of public hospitals due to the pressures of the reform era, thereby tying patients' hands in addressing their medical disputes. Other channels, such as the CCA, had limited power and ability to influence hospitals due to the decentralization and horizontal fragmentation of various ministries (Mertha, 2005). With limited and ineffective institutional channels for addressing their grievances, increased disputes and disruptive actions targeting hospitals were foreseeable in the 2000s.

2.2 A Fragmented Medical Dispute Resolution Landscape in the Transition Era

As discussed, the old health malpractice regulation system was criticized for protecting the interests of health institutions and leaving citizens limited room to protect their rights. Hence, in 2002, the new medical malpractice regulation was promogulated, and a series of changes occurred. First, the new regulation shifted the burden of proof to health institutions to better align with patients' interests.[9] Meanwhile, to avoid conflicts of interest between health institutions and hospitals in technical medical examinations, the new regulation allowed patients to petition higher- or national-level medical associations, believed to be more neutral and objective. More crucially, the scope for medical malpractice was broadened to include any injuries or damages (not limited to death or major injury) related to medical negligence, even if not directly caused by medical malpractice (Wang & Oliphant, 2012). The amended regulation placed more pressure on health institutions, forcing them to improve medical quality and prevent malpractice. However, the new regulation failed to win the support of the healthcare professionals and decrease malpractice cases. According to Guangzhou Health Bureau officials, hospitals complained that the high compensation levels were not proportional to the existing low medical service fees and high risks in the health industry.[10] A grassroots saying emerged: "To get rich,

---

[8] "Brief profiles of spokespersons of ministries of the State Council", The Chinese journalist 8 (1994): 42–43.

[9] See, for instance, medical malpractice regulation (2002), https://www.gov.cn/gongbao/content/2002/content_61445.htm, accessed on September 17, 2023.

[10] See, for instance, The substantial increase in compensation standards in the new medical malpractice regulations has attracted the attention of all parties, http://fzggw.cq.gov.cn/zwxx/bmdt/202002/t20200212_5201205_wap.html, accessed on September 17, 2023.

do the surgery, sue the hospital first, then the doctor (要致富 做手术 告完医院 告大夫)."

While the amended regulations put vulnerable citizens in a better position to protect their rights, the legal channels remained ineffective, time-consuming, and incompetent, frustrating many citizens (He, 2009). From 2002 to 2010, the case closure rate for medical malpractice was only 50%.[11] Since the late 1990s, its promotion of the rule of law prompted the Party-state to channel the discontent back to courtrooms. However, the ineffective legal responses to medical malpractice cases and the rising tide of rights protection activities in China in the 2000s made this problematic. Chinese citizens have increasingly used contentious behaviors to negotiate with the local government to realize and prioritize their interests. Especially in rural areas, where grievances are rampant, citizens with limited resources and government connections often realize their written rights and protect their interests through protest tactics and mobilization (Chen, 2009; 2012; O'Brien, 1996; O'Brien & Li, 2006; Michelson, 2007). Likewise, citizens, especially those marginalized or socially and economically disadvantaged, often perceive medical malpractice as a rivalry between the powerless and the powerful. When patients pay for a laundry list of medical services that fail to address their problems, they become angry and feel unfairly treated. Resorting to collective actions or disruptive behaviors is a useful tool for vulnerable citizens with limited resources to arouse the government's immediate response, albeit through law-breaking and disruptive behaviors.

The rise of disturbances and disruptions in hospitals has also been attributed to China's changing political opportunity structure in the transition era. Since the 1990s, despite limited political opportunity, popular contention has become pluralized in China, threatening the legitimacy and stability of the Party-state's governance. Mass incidents and collective actions derived from social conflicts have become major concerns for local rulers. Collective actions jeopardize politicians' careers or promotions and endanger the Party-state's ruling authority and legitimacy. In dealing with the rise in collective actions, Hu Jintao's administration prioritized social stability as the Party-state's primary goal. According to Wang and Minzner (2015), the rise of the Chinese security state has complicated state-society relations, and single government bureaus can no longer handle disputes; rather, an array of government authorities, including police, legal forces, and public institutions, are all involved. Prioritizing social stability maintenance involves multiple institutions, revealing their conflicting interests and goals.

In medical dispute resolution, the conflicts of interest among government, courts, and hospitals arising from fragmented authoritarianism (Fu, 2017a, b; Mertha, 2005) also unexpectedly encouraged citizens with social grievances to utilize disruptive actions to prioritize their interests. From the government's perspective, the Hu-wen governance reshaped local cadres' behaviors by prioritizing social stability. Due to cadre promotion incentives, local cadres greatly discouraged collective actions,

---

[11] See, for instance, Balance the interests of both doctors and patients and properly handle medical disputes, http://rmfyb.chinacourt.org/paper/images/2010-01/14/08/2010011408_pdf, accessed on September 17, 2023.

especially avoiding collective actions and skip-level petitioning. To maintain social stability and restore order quickly (Chen, 2017; Wang, 2015) local governments often over-compensated when dealing with medical disputes involving collective actions, currying patients' favor in exchange for social stability. While this disadvantaged hospitals, local courts were also under pressure to maintain stability. This new "stability over all" phenomenon exposed the conflicts of interest between government authorities, giving ordinary citizens a political opportunity to use rightful resistance to realize their interests, leading to a wave of hospital violence.

For instance, on 18 June 2009, in Nanping City, Fujian Province (southern China), 50-year-old Yang Junbin (杨俊斌) died during a common percutaneous nephrolithotomy (surgical removal of kidney stones). The whole Yang Village was shocked by their clan member's sudden death, and aggrieved villagers flocked to the hospital. Per existing medical dispute regulations, the hospital communicated with the Yang family, tried to seal the medical records, and recommended an autopsy. However, the Yang clan ascribed the death to the doctors' carelessness and arrogance, becoming even more agitated when one doctor addressed them as "country folk". Fifty angry villagers occupied the hospital, forced the doctor to kneel before the dead body, and demanded compensation. Yang Chun'en, the village head, justified their behaviors:

> We are all farmers and do not understand or believe the 'big' theory you told us. We would not go for the medical technical examination as the involved medical professors are all standing on the hospital's side. How could we trust you? The patient died in your hospital, so you must compensate the family.[12]

Feeling neglected and belittled by the hospital and its doctors, the villagers publicly expressed their anger, helplessness, and distrust, using collective actions to prioritize their pursuit, address their concerns, and be taken seriously. The Yang villagers' deep sadness, shared social connections, anger, and internal solidarity fueled their collective actions and provided moral meaning and justification for their violent behaviors. After the incident, Yang's son posted a gratitude letter[13] praising the Yang villagers' acts of justice (申张正义) on the front door of the house.

The case in Nanping was far from unusual; "failure to address civil disputes" often breeds social unrest in the 2000s (Cai, 2008, p. 108). In one city in eastern China, a collective action against a hospital started out small, when the wife of a construction worker suffered a miscarriage in a famous tertiary hospital. This bad news spread quickly among fellow migrant workers, resonating with their frustrations of being strangers in a strange city. Aiming to "find justice" for their fellow worker, more than a hundred discontented migrant workers occupied the hospital, turning the social conflict into a large-scale mass incident.[14] Given the rise of disturbances in

---

[12] See, for instance, Tang and Liu, Case of Nanping: Health Ecology in China, *China Newsweek*, (22 August 2014), https://np.fjsen.com/2014-08/25/content_14753680_all.htm, accessed on September 17, 2023.

[13] *Ibid.*

[14] Interview with a government officer in C city in August 2016.

public institutions, hospital violence was listed as a new category of mass incidents since 2010 (Du, 2015).[15]

With collective actions against hospitals surging, local officials, rather than judges and legal workers, played a critical role in dealing with medical disputes. Many local government officials, pressured to ensure social stability, made a radical shift from protecting hospitals to favoring individuals. For instance, in the Yang case, local officials "overlooked" violent acts like kidnapping, insults, and threats and took no further actions to stop angry patients. After the violence (facilitated by local government officials) took place, the Nanping Hospital still had to provide 210,000 yuan to compensate the Yang family, without further technical medical examination.[16] The officials later explained their "inactivity" in dealing with the violence, saying that the working protocol for resolving medical disputes in Fujian province (2009) required them to:

> Disperse the crowd; do not force them to be together (可散不可聚);
>
> Solve problems; do not make them even worse (可解不可结);
>
> Do not irritate the people; show kindness to the people (可顺不可激).[17]

Local officials do not want to bring trouble upon themselves, and the working protocol was drafted under the principle of doing everything possible to "maintain political and social stability". Since 2002, social stability has become the primary veto indicator in measuring local government performance. Local governments often make concessions to avoid blame and trouble and prevent incidents from escalating. Since collective actions targeting hospitals do not threaten local governments' legitimacy, they avoid getting involved or using police to intervene, which was often taken as the hospitals' "umbrella of protection". One government interviewee commented, "It is tough to tell right from wrong in these types of medically related cases. We are not experts; what we can do is to separate them physically."[18] Driven by blame avoidance, local governments seldom use forceful interventions in cases of hospital violence, putting hospitals' tranquility at risk. Government officials' "tolerance" offered incentives for the frequent use of disruptive actions targeting hospitals in dispute resolution. However, governments' "laissez-faire" attitudes often backfire. For instance, the next day after the Yang case, medical workers in the hospital adopted similar tactics, flooding the streets to express their discontent to the local government.

Hence, hospitals' interests have been undermined to accommodate patients' disruptive actions and local governments' blame-avoidance mindsets. In exchange for peace, hospitals frequently negotiate privately with patients to settle medical disputes through monetary exchange to discourage collective actions. For instance, from 2006

---

[15] See, for instance, Zhichun Du, Advances in China Public Security, Internal report, 2015.

[16] See, for instance, Hundreds of doctors in Fujian sit in: Still forced to pay compensation after being beaten, http://news.sina.com.cn/c/sd/2009-07-01/113418131379.shtml, accessed on September 17, 2023.

[17] See, for instance, Emergency Disposal Protocol for Mass Incidents in Fujian 2009 Policy No. 266, internal document.

[18] Interview with the public security officer in the C city, September 2016.

to 2007, there were 554 medical disputes in Nanping City alone, with patients receiving total compensation of 11.71 million yuan[19]; hospital violence against healthcare professionals also rose. Similarly, a single district in Shanghai provided 8.5 million yuan in monetary compensation from 2006 to 2008. Li and Deng (2015) estimated that compensation paid by public hospitals in medical disputes exceeded 7.5 billion yuan in 2014 (equivalent to 0.2% of total national health expenditure).

At the same time, the courtrooms were also subject to stability maintenance demands and popular pressure, though only 20%[20] of medical disputes were resolved through legal channels. For instance, on 25 July 2001, Gao Shang (高尚), the son of a deceased patient grieving the loss of his father, attacked a doctor with a glass frame, causing a minor injury.[21] Gao explained that the attack was an accident during a quarrel. On 7 August 2001, he was arrested and faced a civil lawsuit demanding 60,000 RMB compensation.[22] The case, though not a medical dispute, attracted wide media, public, and government attention. The People's Congress representative attended the trial, and the deputy director of the Ministry of Health's Department of Medical Affairs visited the doctor to express his condolences. The case aroused a heated public debate. Some professionals supported the doctor and agreed that Gao should be punished in court, while other ordinary bystanders sympathized with Gao, arousing empathy for his loss. As Gao's mother said, "I was on the edge of collapse for losing my husband and witnessing my son in prison. However, I also received the people's sympathy and righteousness support. I think the law should not bully the weak".[23] Public sympathy for the patient's family and pressure from professional groups put the trial at stake. The court had to balance public perceptions of morality and empathy with the interests of professionals.

Liebman (2013) suggested that China's formal legal system operates in the shadow of protest and violence. Facing popular pressure, courts often judge medical malpractice cases not merely on technical medical examinations but also on political concerns for stability maintenance. Hospitals sometimes offer patients no-fault compensation to address social grievances and avoid escalating disruptive behaviors. According to the People's Court newspaper, cases involving no-fault compensation (无责补偿) increased from 10.8% in 2002 to 25.4% in 2007 (Sun et al., 2010). To some extent,

---

[19] See, for instance, The two-year compensation amount of all hospitals in Nanping is as high as 11.71 million, http://news.sina.com.cn/c/sd/2009-07-01/113418131379_4.shtml, accessed on September 17, 2023.

[20] See, for instance, Beijing Evening News (aaaaaaasffgfgffddsA2001) The violent incident in the Peking Union Medical College Hospital continues: Only 20% of doctor-patient disputes are brought to court, http://news.sina.com.cn/s/2001-07-28/314791.html, accessed on September 17, 2023.

[21] See, for instance, The trial of the attack on a doctor at Peking Union Medical College Hospital was held and NPC deputies attended, http://news.sina.com.cn/c/2001-12-06/413742.html, accessed on September 17, 2023.

[22] See, for instance, The beating of Xiehe doctor continues: The doctor who beat him was formally arrested, http://news.sina.com.cn/c/2001-08-07/322883.html, accessed on September 17, 2023.

[23] See, for instance, The wound was 2 centimeters long after three court sessions? The case became more and more bizarre as the trial progressed, http://news.sina.com.cn/c/2002-03-11/1451503657.html, accessed on September 17, 2023.

courts also used monetary compensation in exchange for social stability and to avoid collective actions. Consequently, in the 2000s, the legal and political systems' institutional constraints made the dispute resolution channel fragmented, ineffective, and subordinate to stability maintenance.

In short, under Hu-wen's reign, institutional responses to social disputes were fragmented. Although China is known for its high state capacity and power, vertical and horizontal fragmentation among government authorities is widespread (Mertha, 2005; Fu, 2017a; Qiaoan, 2020). Ambiguity in assigning responsibility for these new social disputes has led to fragmented governance and blame-avoidance mindsets among various institutions. In dealing with medical disputes, the fragmented and conflicting horizontal interests across such departments as courts, local government, and public hospitals have given citizens the political opportunity to maneuver and apply disruptive actions to realize personal interests and protect their rights. The government aimed to contain all collective actions to avoid regime threats (Hildebrant, 2013), while courts and hospitals aimed to protect the authority of the law and professionals; thus, political stability pressures shrouded the medical dispute resolution process during the 2000s.

2.3 Integrated Stability Maintenance Mechanism

2.3.1 Evolved Social Stability Mechanism

Since President Xi assumed office, the Party-state has attached great importance to social stability maintenance, albeit through refashioned, evolving strategies and institutions. Under his governance, the number of hospital violence has decreased nationwide. For instance, from 2014 to 2018, violent cases dropped from 263 to 57 in Guangzhou, a province heavily struck by hospital violence incidents.[24] Today, social stability maintenance has evolved in many facets. First, resorting to the rule of law instead of violent repression, the government has institutionalized legal weapons to criminalize citizens' disruptive behaviors in social disputes. For instance, the Criminal Procedure Law of China (Article 291),[25] promulgated in 2015, is considered the first law to criminalize hospital violence. According to the law, when disruptive behaviors in health institutions cause serious losses, ringleaders shall be sentenced to fixed-term imprisonment of between three and seven years; other active participants shall be sentenced to three years imprisonment, criminal detention, or deprivation of political rights. In fact, the Chinese government has applied stability justice as an alternative tool for managing petitioning activities to maintain social stability and

[24] See, for instance, Guangdong successfully mediated 11,094 medical disputes in 9 years and the number of hospital violence cases dropped, http://www.xinhuanet.com/politics/2019-11/16/c_1125239362.htm, accessed on September 18, 2023.

[25] See, for instance, Criminal Procedure Law of the People's Republic of China, http://www.npc.gov.cn/zgrdw/englishnpc/Law/2007-12/13/content_1384067.htm, accessed on September 18, 2023.

governance legitimacy. For instance, Feng and Zeng (2022) found that petitioner defendants are more likely to be detained before a politically sensitive period to avoid disruptive or collective actions. Legal weapons are applied to deter citizens from applying disruptive actions and collective actions to protect their rights. It has also given local governors a legal basis for penalizing and punishing law-breaking behaviors in hospitals and an alternative to repressive measures.

Second, the timing of government interventions has been moved forward in a preventive manner, shifting from sporadic crisis management to the paradigm of "source governance" (to address the dispute from the origin, 源头治理; see also Hu & Wu, 2023). More efforts have focused on source governance and preventing social disputes to nip hidden dangers in the bud. Advanced technologies and more human resources are employed to identify potential petitioners and channel them to official institutions, such as local courts, to achieve reconciliation before petitioning activities occur. For instance, digital measures like big data and the Internet have been used to not only identify potential risks precisely and routinely, but also promote coordination between various departments. Maintaining social stability has become more routinized and institutionalized rather than only being applied during a crisis or sensitive period. According to Ma Yusheng (马玉生), deputy director of the central stability maintenance office (中央维稳办), "the idea of social stability needs to be refashioned. It is like preventive medicine. When the collective action occurs, regardless of how properly it is managed, the damage and influence is irresistible, and the cost is much higher than preventing."[26]

Third, the stability maintenance mechanism has become more institutionalized and integrated, replacing the fragmented governance derived from conflicts of interest among various institutions. In 2014, prioritizing social order, Xi called for a joint effort from all of society to maintain social stability and order.[27] Xi criticized the indifferent attitudes in dealing with citizens' grievances and promoted a more proactive, integrated dispute resolution mechanism by increasing responsiveness to bottom-up demands. Adhering to the "horizontal to the edge, vertical in the end" logic (*hengxiang daobian zongxiang daodi* 横向到边, 纵向到底),[28] this system involves joint actions by various political authorities to maintain social stability. The priority of stability maintenance is well-aligned as long as one belongs to the government system. Previously, the primary responsibility rested with the Public Security Bureau,

---

[26] See, for instance, "Fight the initiative to maintain stability under the new situation—In-depth study of Comrade Xi Jinping's important exposition on maintaining overall social stability", https://china.huanqiu.com/article/9CaKrnJZHZ3, accessed on September 18, 2023.

[27] See, for instance, Xi Jinping attended the Central Political and Legal Work Conference and delivered an important speech, http://cpc.people.com.cn/n/2014/0109/c64094-24065903.html, accessed on September 18, 2023.

[28] This strategy implies that the entire stability maintenance system should encompass top formal institutions to grassroots institutions as well as extending horizontally from core departments to peripheral departments to maintain stability. For example, see ZhenJingming, 'zongxiangdaodi, hengxiangdaobian' ['horizontal to the edge, vertical in the end'], *Guangming Daily,* (9 December 2006), available at: http://www.gmw.cn/01gmrb/2006-12/09/content_519913.htm, accessed on September 18, 2023.

and expenditures on public security increased annually due to the increasing danger and occurrence of grassroots conflicts and collective actions (Yan, 2016). However, many other departments are in the social stability maintenance chain of command today, including the juridical department, local government, and the grassroots community. For instance, in dealing with hospital violence, the government promoted collaboration between hospital and police authorities to deter law-breakers, known as the "police-doctor partnership" (警医联动). Routinized procedures and protocols were established to prevent and deal with bottom-up crises. Through broadened participation, an integrated, all-encompassing social stability maintenance mechanism has been established to supervise all social disputes and threats to social stability.

Among the integrated stability maintenance mechanisms, a new-yet-old institution—people's mediation—is noteworthy, as it plays a central role in connecting various government authorities, addressing disputes, and nipping social instability in the bud. Since Xi took power, he has been keen on recalling traditional Maoist institutions to address emerging social problems. As Xi commented, "the condition of China determined that we cannot become the litigation country. We should give priority to the non-litigation dispute settlement mechanism. Social disputes should be addressed at the grassroots level through the role of mediation. It would make our grassroots community more harmonious and stable, as the basis for building a Peaceful China."[29] From the institutional perspective, repurposing traditional mediation institutions has reduced the sunk cost of starting from scratch (Genschel, 1997) and minimized political risks by averting the escalation of social disputes, preventing regime change and enhancing the regime's information collection capacity. Mediation institutions, which absorb and deal with social disputes through their daily practices, have contributed to the regime's grassroots stability. For instance, special people's mediation committees, including medical dispute mediation committees, are created to address disputes in professional fields, redirecting citizens' grievances to the institutionalized channel.

Meanwhile, the people's mediation institutions also act as a transmission belt linking various institutions. For instance, according to the *People's Mediation Law* passed in 2010,[30] local courts and police authorities could channel dispute cases to the people's mediation institutions (Article 18). During mediation, mediators must report sensitive cases to police authorities and other departments, take preventive strategies, and avoid escalating disputes (Article 25). In other words, the people's mediation institutions have become central to social stability maintenance, connecting juridical, policing, and grassroots forces. The law addressed the conflicts of interest and blame-avoidance mindsets among various institutions by taking the initiative in dispute resolution, and is now applied to address medical disputes as wicked social problems.

[29] See, for instance, Xi Jinping: Unswervingly follow the path of socialist rule of law with Chinese characteristics and provide strong legal guarantee for the comprehensive construction of a modern socialist country, http://www.xinhuanet.com/politics/2021-02/28/c_1127149742.htm, accessed on September 18, 2023.

[30] See, for instance, People's Mediation Law of the Peoples' Republic of China, https://www.gov.cn/flfg/2010-08/29/content_1691209.htm, accessed on September 18, 2023.

As such, China has developed a high level of resilience to maintain social and political order.

2.3.2 *Institutional Change in People's Mediation Institutions in China*

Gandhi and Przeworski (2007) stated that institutions matter in authoritarian regimes. Recent scholarship has paid increasing attention to institutions under authoritarianism, especially how they structure political power, organize political representation, and facilitate regime sustainability (Pepinksy, 2014; Boix & Svolik, 2013; Svolik, 2008; Slater, 2003). This chapter traces and examines the institutional change of China's people's mediation institutions, a political and socially distinctive institution featuring Party traditions and cutting-edge adaptive characteristics. People's mediation institutions refer to government-sponsored dispute resolution institutions with government-embedded personnel efforts established to promote mutual understanding and reconciliation between disputants, satisfying both the social management and social control goals at the grassroots. Unlike in Western societies, where mediation channels are primarily carried out by a third party, people's mediation is deeply embedded in China's social and political institutions. Rather, the Chinese government invested heavily in the building of the people's mediation to solicit grassroots support and maintain social order. The vitality of the people's mediation lies in the strong adaptability to the changing social and political landscape from the 1930s till now.

The history of the people's mediation can be traced back to the Revolutionary Era. In the revolutionary era, new problems produced by the new lifestyle, such as free marriage and land disputes, placed a heavy burden on grassroots government. During this, Ma Xiwu, a revolutionist, created a new model of adjudication to increase the efficiency of dispute resolution, consolidate power, and enhance grassroots legitimacy. Instead of following rules and regulations inflexibly, Ma Xiwu's approach considered cultural contexts and public opinion, exercising political persuasion with disputants' consent and for their satisfaction. Mao praised and promoted Ma Xiwu's way of adjudication, which involves roving tribunals convened in rural communities, combining mediation and litigation as an alternative approach to ease the burden on local courts, following the mass line (Cong, 2014). Mediation institutions' political roles were also evident. Through intermediary roles such as Ma, the Communist Party successfully filled the social power void at the grassroots level caused by replacing the old social gentry, while realizing social control in rural communities.

The mediation tradition persisted after the CPC's 1949 victory. As Mao praised in 1958, "Ma Xiwu's method is suitable for civil dispute resolution by conducting investigation and research, prioritizing mediation, and solving the dispute right on the spot."[31] The reasons for institutionalizing mediation channels are numerous. First, their advent efficiently constrained the scope of civil disputes by providing immediate responses at the grassroots level, avoiding the escalation of disputes and lawsuits. Second, the mediation channel helped maintain social relations at the grassroots level in the regime's early years. According to Xie Juezai (谢觉哉), then president of the People's Supreme Court, the mediation channel better maintained harmonious social relations in rural areas and saved labor by reducing big problems to a manageable size.[32] For instance, there once was a fight between a local family and a disabled veteran in Yan'an because of the quarrel over lending furniture. Xie visited the local family and explained to the villager the difficult situation of the disabled veteran. He expressed his apology on behalf of the veteran. The local family was touched. Xie later visited the local government and freed the veteran from further punishment. Mass persuasion and seeking disputants' consent were effective in dispute resolution, which also restored the harmonious relations at the grassroots and prevented the use of legal sanctions. Third, mediation institutions followed the Party's long-pursued mass-line strategy, complementing traditional legal responses to enable vulnerable social groups to articulate their interests and express their grievances, enhancing local cadres' information collection role and identifying emergent problems. It also reflected the Party-state's benevolent governance by being responsive to ordinary citizens, enhancing the regime's moral legitimacy. Hence, by the end of 1955, mediation institutions were well-established in 70% of neighborhoods and rural communities across China (Wang, 1985).

By the end of 1981, after being disbanded during the Cultural Revolution, mediation institutions were widely restored and re-established in rural and urban communities and work unit systems. The number of mediators also had grown from one million in 1955 to 4.7 million in 1981 (Wang, 1985). In 1981 alone, twelve times as many cases (mainly interpersonal disputes) went through mediation channels than legal channels. Mediation avoided the escalation of social conflict between citizens and contributed to the solidarity of the masses.

However, the legitimacy of mediation institutions has faced significant shortfalls and challenges in the transition era. Since the reform and opening up and the increased law and rule consciousness among citizens (Perry, 2008), the role of people's mediation has declined. For instance, according to Xiong Yihan's fieldnote (2006) from an interview with established mediator Yang Boshou,

> From 1994 to 1998, the mediation institutions could not issue written agreements among the disputants, but only verbal promises. Since mediation is not legally binding, causing low credibility, people often prefer to go to court. Even the mediators themselves also proactively channeled and encouraged the disputants to the court, which is the same practice among the police and residence committee also did the same. In 1998, the cadre from the Supreme Court

[31] See, for instance, Coordination and Enlightenment of "Mediation Relationship" in Shaanxi-Gansu-Ningxia Border Region. http://www.rmfyb.com/paper/html/2013-11/08/content_72539.htm?div=-1, accessed on September 18, 2023.

[32] See, for instance, Harmony in the countryside, saving labor for production . http://dangshi.people.com.cn/n1/2016/0202/c85037-28104463.html, accessed on September 18, 2023.

commented, 'people's mediation as the flower of the Oriental has faded away.' (Xiong, 2006; p.101–102).

The critical juncture occurred at the beginning of the 2000s. Mediation institutions' retreat prompted the Party-state to adopt legal and extra-legal approaches (policing, letter-and-visit bureaus, administrative adjuncts, etc.) to deal with the rise in grassroots disputes. The end of the work unit system and the mediation committees' decline pushed disputants into the courtroom. However, these legal and extra-legal channels failed to respond to citizens' grievances effectively and efficiently, sometimes leading to dispute escalation and collective actions. As such, in September 2002, China's Supreme Court promulgated the *Regulation on the Civil Cases Involving People's Mediation Agreement*,[33] which gave legal authority to mediation agreements as civil contracts. In addition, the Supreme Court proposed "more mediation less jurisdiction" (能调则调, 多调少判) as a guideline for social dispute resolution to ease the burden on heavily-loaded courtrooms and accelerate the dispute resolution process, connecting the people's and court mediation channels. According to the then-president of the Supreme Court, Xiao Yang (肖扬), the courts should confirm agreements reached through people's mediation channels to avoid and reduce litigation pressure and ease demands on juridical resources.[34] By directing cases to mediation institutions, the case closure rate through the mediation channel climbed above 32% from 2000 to 2004.[35]

The return of mediation could be understood through the lens of the retreat of the rule of law in China. Since the 1990s, the Party-state's rule-of-law reforms have modernized the state but mobilized citizens to adopt the law to protect their interests directly against public institutions and the state (Gallagher, 2006), generating many social grievances and disputes. Specifically, courts have been "dysfunctional" in dealing with the growing pains of Chinese citizens in the transitional era (Zhuang & Chen, 2015; Hu, 2011). Zero-sum litigation often mobilizes unsatisfied disputants to undertake disruptive actions and repeatedly petition higher courts and the government to realize their interests. The overwhelming caseload also faces legal workers' judicial incompetence and courts' inability (Peerenboom & He, 2009). In the 2010s, overwhelmed by rocketing disputes and stability concerns, the Party-state decided to turn away from the courts and adopt the traditional Maoist tool of people's mediation to realize dispute resolution and restore social order. In a sense, the Party-state intended mediation institutions to "replace" courts and restore social stability and dispute resolution.

---

33 See, for instance, Several provisions of the supreme people's court on the trial of civil cases involving people's mediation agreements policy consultation, http://fgcx.bjcourt.gov.cn:4601/law?fn=chl253s072.txt&term=1, accessed on September 18, 2023.

34 See, for instance, Xiao Yang: Give full play to the positive role of judicial mediation in building a harmonious society, https://www.gov.cn/govweb/jrzg/2006-10/06/content_405961.htm, accessed on September 18, 2023.

35 See, for instance, Create a new situation in the grassroots construction of people's courts, http://gongbao.court.gov.cn/Details/6ad0af46bbc1c41cf9f020b32d8fbd.html, accessed on September 18, 2023.

The revival of people's mediation reflected a Chinese-style understanding of justice and the rule of law. People's mediation merged Chinese Confucianism with communist genes, reflecting the revival of the mass line strategy to address social disputes. Public perceptions of justice largely depend on the system's outcomes and efficacy. If it contains only legal norms, not social norms like favor, face, and social power, it will fail to satisfy public expectations of justice, often leading to repetitive petitions. Professor Zhu Suli (朱苏力), from the Law School of Peking University, noted that "we now focused on procedure justice too much, which I do not oppose. However, the substantial justice still matters. The procedure protected the interests of a judge, not the disputants. ...We must balance procedural and substantial justice to satisfy the social demands."[36] Unlike legal channels, mediation involves the innovative appliance of legal and social norms through mass involvement in judgement and intensive fieldwork. It is less bound by rules, can be flexibly applied to address social disputes, and can better align with Party interests while satisfying public expectations of justice and appearing effective.

In addition to political leaders' promotion, from a bottom-up perspective, revitalizing people's mediation represented the interests of local governments. Mediation channels allow the local government to address the disputes more flexibly, satisfying the interests of local bureaucrats. Zhuang Wenjia and Chen Feng (2015) examined the rationales behind the revival of mediation in labor dispute resolution at the local and state level. Economically, promoting mediation could afford governments discretionary power and limit economic compensation, compared to strictly adhering to the labor compensation standards set by law. Politically, mediation better aligns with local governments' need to maintain social stability by avoiding labor protests and other mass incidents. Simultaneously, the mediation rate has been linked with performance evaluation by courts and judges (He, 2021), as it is more convenient and efficient for judges to choose mediation over litigation to avoid eliciting appeals. People's mediation channels are a pragmatic Party-state tool that absorbs unaddressed social grievances by accommodating conflicting goals, such as the rule of law, stability maintenance, and economic development.

By promoting mediation, the Party-state has established an all-encompassing social dispute-resolution mechanism that combines various political and social resources. Professor Hu Jieren described it as Grand Mediation, incorporating various governmental resources, including the juridical department, local government, people's mediation, and conflicting parties (Hu, 2011, p. 1071). Mediation is a bridge connecting various government bureaus in the all-encompassing dispute resolution landscape. By co-opting professional and coercive authorities into resolving social disputes, a new model of people's mediation was soon diffused across China.

Today, people's mediation has been gradually patched up with new functions to address various social disputes, including medical disputes involving professional expertise and heightened emotion. It is essential to note that dealing with medical disputes differs from labor and other traditional disputes in several ways. First, the

---

[36] See, for instance, The patterns of Chinese justice, http://cdfy.scssfw.gov.cn/article/detail/2009/12/id/571857.shtml, accessed on September 18, 2023.

disputants involved in medical disputes are more diverse: some are uneducated, some are resourceful, some are interest-driven, and some are in a deep grievance, while almost all of them are hard to reach reconciliation. Meanwhile, the responsibility attribution of medical disputes is still ambiguous. During the fieldwork, I found that disputants are often hostile and have the natural inclination to distrust the hospitals, hence many are reluctant to perform the medical technical examination. To some extent, the dispute resolution was carried out in the environment without the clear cut of right and wrong. Third, under deep grievance, the disputants often hold high expectations towards the compensation of medical disputes, which makes the mediation process even harder. For instance, in the city, one family raised the proposal of one million RMB compensation (equivalent to 145,000 USD) for the death of a patient who committed suicide in the hospital. Driven by such high monetary expectations, it often costs mediators large efforts to perform reconciliation and persuasion between two parties.

Thus, puzzles arise, how do the mediators persuade the disputants in the medical dispute resolution which seems to be a mission impossible? Extant studies often examine the rise of mediation from the institutional perspective, yet few investigate the mechanism of mediation and the embedded distributive logic of the mediation. Before moving to the following chapters, the next section first theorized the institutional constraints of the mediators which provided the base for politicized dispute resolution in China.

2.4 Institutional Constraints of Mediation Institutions and Politicalized Outcomes

Patients use legal weapons to sue the hospitals and doctors through court litigation, which is time-consuming, expensive, and has an uncertain outcome (Studdert et al., 2006). Hence, in many legal studies, mediation is a common approach to settle social disputes as an alternative dispute resolution (ADR) channel compared to courts context ((Hyman et al., 2010; Liebman & Hyman, 2004; Tena-Tamayo & Sotelo, 2005; Yee, 2005). For instance, according to Liebman and Hyman (2004), mediation is

> "(A)n informal, private, voluntary and confidential process in which a neutral third party- the mediator—helps the participants negotiate their differences and craft a mutually acceptable resolution to their dispute or decide to deal with their problems in some other manner, including litigation. (Liebman & Hyman, 2004, p. 29)".

However, unlike the mediations carried out by the neutral third party, people's mediation in China are a quasi-government institution that is subjected to multi-dimensional institutional constraints, including political, social, and legal concerns. Though many studies examined the rise of mediation applied in labor conflict, the literature remained fragmented. The underlined logic and efficacy of mediation institutions remained unknown and rarely systematically examined. In specific, we are unclear about what institutional constraints and incentives shaped the outcomes and process of the mediation process. In this book, I examine how people's mediation addresses medical disputes by examining its underlined calculation logic.

The people's mediation institutions are embedded under a series of social, political and legal norms. According to the People's Mediation Law,[37] the guiding principle and goals for the people's mediation in dispute resolution is 1) adhering to the principle of law, 2) being based on equity and voluntarily; 3) maintaining the harmony and stability of the society. **First,** adhering to the "principle of law" or "law-binding" means that the dispute resolution process needs to be based on the law, regulation, and policy. The principle confirmed the quasi-legal status of the people's mediation committees. However, it is by no means that we should equate people's mediation with the court, nor does every mediation solution need to follow the procedures and rules unchangeably and consistently. Rather, it pinpoints that the mediation outcome carries legal weight and should not conflict with existing law; while for many uncovered blind spots in the law, the mediation committee could judge based on the socialist-style code of moral ethics and social norms as a substitute to more efficiently address citizens' grievances. The pragmatic attitudes of the mediation institutions aimed to fill the vacuum of uncovered arenas of legal channels and promoted a sense of efficacy through the mediation channel through their own practices of the rule of law.

Second, the principle of equity and voluntarily emphasized that the mediation should be free of coercion, threat, and repression, and need to be merely based on the disputants' willingness voluntarily. It is very crucial as it implies that citizens' agency and willingness play a decisive role to reach reconciliation in dispute resolution, regardless of how powerful the other disputant party is. Since many disputants involved in mediation is vulnerable (Michelson, 2007), the introduction of the mediation committees aims to change the power asymmetry between vulnerable citizen and powerful private institution (such as hospitals or private companies). Introducing the mediators into the dispute resolution process, helped individual disputants gain more bargaining power by adding more weight to citizens' side. However, since the mediation institutions are government-sponsored and the mediators as public personnel, they could be never free from political influence or personal effect. Thus, the social power game during the mediation process is also not evitable.

Third, political considerations are amongst the most institutional constraints in shaping the way people's mediation works and the outcomes of mediation. As discussed, the Party-state has been increasingly concerned about building a harmonious society and maintaining social stability. The political stability concern has been reflected in many facets of the People's Mediation Law. For instance, as stated in Article 21 of the People's Mediation Law, the mediators should prevent the escalation of conflict timely manner to confine the disputes locally (及时、就地进行).[38] The government therefore depends on the mediation channels to achieve a social control

[37] See, for instance, People's Mediation Law of the Peoples' Republic of China, https://www.gov.cn/flfg/2010-08/29/content_1691209.htm, accessed on September 18, 2023.

[38] *Ibid.*

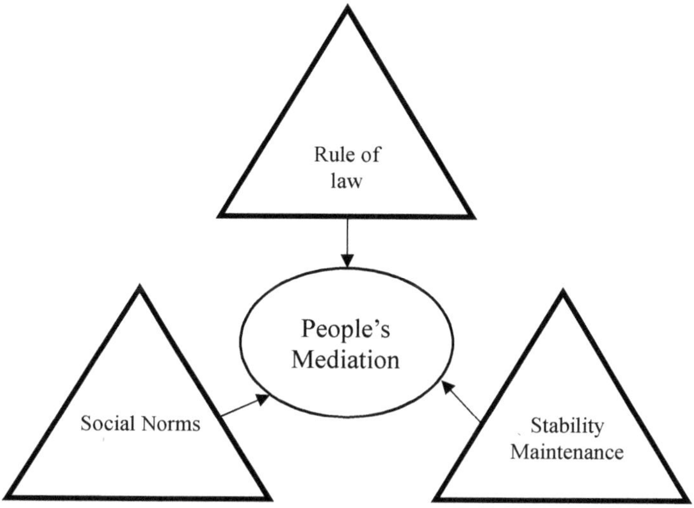

Fig. 2.1 The institutional foundations of people's mediation

role (Zhou, 2023) by depending on the capacity of the mediators and freeing themselves from being directly involved in dispute resolution. Taken together, I argue that the people's mediation is in the integration and dynamic interactions of the rule of law, social power, and stability maintenance (See Fig. 2.1). The process and results of medical dispute resolution in China are influenced by the dynamic interaction between legal, social power, and political factors.

2.4.1 *Rule of Law*

Rule of law emphasized that all the procedures and outcomes of the mediation shall follow the procedures and rules, and are legally bound. Among the first pillar, adhering to the law not only enables the results of the mediation to be legally effective but also makes the mediation a part of the formal element in the juridical system in China. According to the People's Mediation Law launched in 2010,

> "(A)ll parties shall perform as agreed. After the mediation is reached through the mediation, if necessary, they may jointly apply to the People's Court for judicial confirmation within thirty days from the day when the mediation agreement takes effect. Once the People's Court confirms the validity of the mediation agreement in accordance with the law, if one party refuses to perform or fails to fully perform, the other party may apply to the People's Court for compulsory execution." (Article 31, Article 33).

As mediation institutions have gradually become a part of the formal legal institutions, they have become increasingly cautious about managing and facilitating the mediation process by playing by the rules. On the one hand, it could help the mediation institutions gain formality and professionalism to increase organizational legitimacy by showing respect to the existing rules, procedures, and regulations. In other words, anyone who violated the outcome would be considered a violator, which constrains citizens' behaviors and promotes them to follow the mediation's outcomes. On the other hand, the principle of the rule of law did not refrain the mediation institutions from utilizing discretionary power. Instead, the mediation channels could muddle through the grey zones that have been uncovered by the rules. The revitalization of the people's mediation committees provided the political space for mediators to address the disputes flexibly. For instance, in dealing with family disputes, the mediators not only merely mediate based on law or regulations only, instead, they often shift their focus from conflicts to providing love and care for their children in order to make the divorcing couple reconcile and preserve social harmony. People's mediation committees could employ both formal and informal practices under the name of rule of law to readdress the social disputes. It showed how the Party-state has been sophisticated enough to apply the rule of law strategically to social governance and achieve the social control goal through upholding the law strategically.

Through the mediation channel, the mediation often put equal blame on the put parties and adopt extra-legal rules to achieve the reconciliation between disputants. The "plastering over" style of mediation used to be considered contradicting with the rule of law, from some legal experts' perspective (Ji, 1989). Since the 1990s, the Party-state has promoted the "rule of law" to regulate the state-society relations, as a part of the state modernization project. However, today, the mediation institution is the fundamental element in the formal legal system. It is partially because in dealing with social disputes, strictly following the existing rules sometimes was conflict with the interests of the local state. For instance, according to Zhuang Wenjia and Chen Feng's (2015),

> They (local state) have strong incentives to depress workers' claims for compensation or to limit the amount of compensation required by the law, and mediation serves this purpose. Local labor bureaus, for instance, rarely apply legal sanctions when handling workers' complaints about employers' breaches of the law as they are afraid that this may hamper business.

Following the rule of law selectively and strategically would better improve the efficiency of the mediation institutions in dispute resolution. Though the mediators are the laymen in the juridical system, they become the gatekeepers in the social dispute resolution process. The introduction of mediation institutions to the formal legal system is to avoid the stubbornness of the legal system by making the legal system more flexible and efficient by incorporating both legal and social norms.

To some extent, revitalization of the mediation did not decrease but helped the local state apply discretional power in cases that are incompatible with the rule to remain flexible in adhering to the "rule of law" principle. By resorting to the mediation channel, the local state could strike the balance between the rule of law and discretional power jointly under the name of the law. For instance, in the arena of medical dispute resolution, the State Council initiated the "regulation on the prevention and handling of medical dispute prevention"[39] in 2018 to regulate the medical dispute resolution process. As the official discourses stated, the mediation agreement should also be in accordance with the socialist morality and code of ethics, providing the political space for the mediation committee to maneuver when the formal regulation could not be applied. Hence, people's mediation which combined the rule of the law and discretional power was flexible to solve the disputes efficiently. It helped the government officials to free themselves from facing criticism and collective actions against the social disputes but also gained legitimacy by redirecting citizens to the mediation. For the grey zone created by the flexible and selective implementation of the rule of law, the local state could utilize mediation as a remedy to produce the government-favored and disputant-satisfied outcomes to solicit the public trust as well. In addition to the formal rules, the mediators also take the informal and implicit rules into account, as the other pillars for the mediation which would be discussed below.

2.4.2 *Social Power: Asymmetric Social Power Between Mediators and Disputants*

The second pillar of mediation lies in the principle of "equality and voluntarily", which requires that the disputants' rights are free of coercion, discrimination, and repressive measures in the mediation process. This is crucial for the mediation process because it indicates that disputants cannot be coercive to reach the resolution, regardless of the authority and power held by the mediators to accelerate the reconciliation process. It implies that the whole mediation process and outcome need voluntary consent from the disputants, and the disputant needs to obey the mediation result voluntarily. However, in practice, power asymmetry and coercion seem inevitable. The asymmetric social power between the mediators and disputants is the key to the mediation process. The mediation process also entails the power interactions between the government-sponsored mediators, public institutions, and vulnerable disputants, which is not void of political influence and social power.

In fact, the process of mediation was under an asymmetric social power influence among the mediators, disputants, and public institutions. The occurrence of social disputes is de facto because of the power asymmetry between the disputants. For instance, the vice deputy of the county-level people's court Liu Xiao suggested that in medical disputes, disadvantaged citizens are more likely to petition and other disruptive behaviors when they find the outcomes of the dispute resolution are biased and favoring public hospitals.[40] The feeling of injustice would motivate powerless

[39] See, for instance, Regulations on the Prevention and Handling of Medical Disputes (2018), https://www.gov.cn/zhengce/content/2018-08/31/content_5318057.htm, accessed on September 18, 2023.

[40] See, for instance, A brief discussion on petitioning issues in medical disputes, https://xpxfy.hncourt.gov.cn/public/detail.php?id=56, accessed on September 18, 2023.

citizens to go to their extreme. When the dispute occurs, the mediators need to analyze the disputants' social ties, connections, and situation, and therefore apply necessary concessions to win their hearts; or assert psychological pressure to accelerate the mediation process. Persuading the disputants through soft strategies, not only addressed the disputes but also changed the disputants' mindsets and comforted their anxiety, which is considered more effective in demobilizing potential collective actions. On the one hand, by utilizing their social influence and authority, the mediators could establish authority over the disputants and limit the severity and scale of the disputes. On the other hand, the vulnerable social power possessed by the disputants also becomes a crucial element for mediators to consider by considering informal rules and eliciting compassion, which leads to a flexible strategy in dealing with social disputes. Hence, the mediation process was also under the power interaction between mediators and disputants.

2.4.2.1 Semi-official Mediators

Mediators involved in social disputes come in a host of forms including social workers, judges, teachers, retired police officers, and other social elites who devoted themselves to dispute resolution. The special identity of the mediators has deeply shaped the way they formulate their messages with the disputant and determined how mediation is carried out.

Since the imperial era, those who got involved in dispute resolution were often the social gentry and full members of villages. They usually shared the same surname with the remaining villagers but held a higher social status and authority due to their education, seniority, and wealth. For instance, Huang's (2008) study found that the government in the Tsing dynasty recruited unsalaried quasi-officials nominated by communities and confirmed by the local government to address disputes. Compared to salaried bureaucrats, these semi-officials could keep down the government burden in a minimalist fashion to avoid government intervention. Through the crucial intermediary role of mediators, it created the "third realm"—an intermediate sphere between the state bureaucracy and society. It greatly contributed to the social governance in the community.

This tradition persisted in contemporary China. According to the policy of "Strengthening the team building of Mediators"[41] issued in 2018,

> "Attention should be paid to recruiting lawyers, arbitrators, grassroots legal workers, doctors, teachers, professors, retired judges, police, and other retired employees in public institutions to take the role of mediators in Peoples' Mediation".

These mediators, as quasi-officials, have natural political ties with the government as most of them have working experiences in the government authorities. Due to their political background, they are familiar with the interests of the local governments

[41] See, for instance, Opinions on strengthening the construction of the team of people's mediators, https://www.gov.cn/xinwen/2018-04/27/content_5286469.htm, accessed on September 18, 2023.

and could the information collection for the governors. Meanwhile, mediators are often deployed and embedded in the community and accumulated authority. Most mediators are recruited by local communities or districts where they reside and work. The social connections with the community entitled them to the higher authority and held them accountable to dispute resolution. As a legacy of tradition, seniority is also a great asset for the mediators. A local official once commented "The ideal age of a mediator is approximately 30–65. If the mediator is too young, it would make himself unreliable among the residents".[42] Hence, the prototypical mediators are believed effective in persuading the disputants and sometimes are the key to dispute resolution.

2.4.2.2 Power of the Weak

If the mediator's characteristics are one factor that shaped the politicization of the mediation process, another crucial factor is the background of the disputants. Some studies identify the correlation between the disputants' socioeconomic background and grievances. For instance, drawing on the data collected in 2002 from 3000 households in various regions in China, Ethan Michelson's study (2007) found that citizens with better resources and political connections are more likely to shield their grievances as they get better access to other solutions. In comparison, grievances and social disputes are often associated with disadvantaged socioeconomic groups. It shaped the moral economy of the dispute resolution in China.

The rise of law consciousness mobilized citizens with a vulnerable social status to shop for venues to address their disputes. A robust literature examined the disputants from relatively vulnerable backgrounds and their dispute resolution channels. The vulnerable background of the disputants could translate to their power in bargaining with the public authorities. In dealing with social disputes, government tends to adopt flexible measures such as mediation, instead of direct repression. Scholars often ascribed the government concession and tolerance to the non-regime-threatening nature of these social disputes. For instance, Cai (2008) ascertained that since some social disputes did not pinpoint the political institutions of socialist regimes, local governments are more likely to tolerate them. In this book, I argue that the social power and moral reasoning of the vulnerable disputants also is one of the pillars that shaped the government and mediators' strategies. In the arena of medical disputes, for instance, the miserable situation and grievances to some extent legitimated their disruptive behaviors and collective actions in the public hospitals. To some extent, holding the doctors or hospitals accountable for the malpractice was considered more "legitimate" and "grounded". The loss of a beloved family member or the deterioration of health often rendered a high degree of grievances and heightened emotions, which provided the justification for the collective actions. For example, as Hurst and O'Brien (2002) stated, "Moral indignation and survival needs are two reasons why pension arrears have so often sparked popular resistance." The hospital violence

[42] Author's fieldnote, in August 2015.

instigated by families is often considered a final resort made by a vulnerable group to seek their "own" justice. Threatening or harassing a doctor may be considered an expression of one's discontent rather than a crime. Hence, medical disputes also represent the moral facet of the popular resistance in China and the mediation process was inevitably shaped by the moral power of the weakness.

Social power concerns required the mediation process to take the social power elements such as the vulnerable status of the disputants into consideration, instead of strictly following the formal rules and guidance. The introduction of the mediators as semi-government officials helped rewrite the power asymmetry that existed between patients and health institutions. Meanwhile, the mediation process is also full of the power interactions between the disputant, hospitals, and mediators. Mediators could be better informed about the social-economic background of the disputants, applying flexible and contingent measures to not only solve the dispute but also establish emotional ties with the disputants. Mediators also could take advantage of their government embeddedness to exert political influence on the hospitals in exchange for their concession. It also suggests the growing and comprehensive capacity of the party-state to manage society and maintain social tranquility by taking social power into consideration.

2.4.3 Political Concern: Stability Maintenance

Today, the people's mediation or Ma Xiwu's style of mediation is widespread in contemporary China. As discussed, like a new wine in an old bottle, people's mediation's roots could be traced back to Maoist characteristics with moralist and populist characteristics which used to be endorsed and praised by Mao for its mass-line strategy. Under Xi's reign, Maoist institutions have often revitalized to address new social problems. The people's mediation, which emerged in the Revolutionary era as a dispute resolution channel, now belonged to a part of the all-encompassing social stability mechanism.

Not surprisingly, the political concern of maintaining social stability is no doubt a founding pillar of the institutional bases for people's mediation institutions. According to the official discourse, people's mediation was the "first line of defense in maintaining social stability" (第一道防线).[43] The mediation process and results need to align with the government's interest in stability maintenance. Mediators shoulder the political responsibility to balance the interests of individuals and groups and to maintain social stability and prevent social disputes from escalating. By intervening in dispute resolution in the earlier stage, it could trace the root of the grievance from its source and collaborate with relevant authorities to deal with the disputes with

[43] See, for instance, Legislation to improve the people's mediation system to build the "first line of defense" for maintaining stability, http://www.npc.gov.cn/zgrdw/huiyi/cwh/1115/2010-06/23/content_1577918.htm, accessed on September 18, 2023.

joint force and therefore maintain stability. Hence, the quest for stability shaped the way the mediators' strategies and mindsets in dealing with medical disputes.

For instance, according to the "indices on mediators' work evaluation" in Jing'an district in Shanghai launched in 2020,[44] the mediators would be added with extra values if they could (1) successfully address the dispute that transferred from local government, (2) resolve collective action that composed of more than three people, and (3) readdress prolonged disputes that have lasted more than five years, with extra two points each (total 10 points as max). In comparison, mediation results that have been revoked or changed by the local courts would be deducted 20 points as a penalty. To maintain social stability, some people's mediation committees have set the goals of "zero petition, zero accident, zero court case" to address bottom-up disputes proactively.

In the arena of medical disputes, maintaining social order also becomes troublesome. The medical dispute involves the loss of lives or severe injuries, which easily could trigger bottom-up collective actions targeting both hospitals and local government. Meanwhile, the pressure of maintaining social order may also come from healthcare professionals. For instance, on 26 August 2014, in Yongzhou, Hunan Province, 200 healthcare professionals protested to the city-level government to request the government protect the rights of medical workers and punish the lawbreakers who created hospital violence one day before.[45] Beyond dispute resolution, mediators also need to identify potential collective actions, relieve the tension between the hospitals and doctors, restore harmonious relations, and increase the sense of satisfaction and efficacy towards the dispute resolution process. The mediation not only addressed the dispute based on the social and legal norms, but the political concerns of stability maintenance also shaped the way, strategy, and timing mediators respond.

2.5 Summary

In summary, this chapter traces the politicization process of the medical dispute resolution in contemporary China. Since the reform and opening up, the social dispute resolution mechanism has shifted from a laissez-faire, and fragmented institutional responses to the all-encompassing social dispute resolution mechanism with the revitalization of the mediation institutions. I argue that the rule of law, asymmetric social power, and the political stability maintenance concerns jointly provided the foundation for the mediation process. This book unveiled the dark box of mediation and examined the everyday politics of mediation. It suggests how politicized medical

[44] See, for instance, Annual Work Assessment Methods for People's Mediators of Jing'an District, Shanghai (Trial), https://www.jingan.gov.cn/govxxgk/JB0/2020-06-29/621bb663-6a8d-4cc0-8b01-7f5ab09582c4.html, accessed on September 19, 2023.

[45] See, for instance, Doctors from Yueyang held a sit-in demanding severe punishment for the murderer, https://www.lifetimes.cn/article/9CaKrnJFtjC, accessed on September 19, 2023.

dispute resolution is shaped by the complex interaction between political, social, and legal concerns. In the following Chapter, I explained why hospital violence takes place in China with limited political space and traced the fragmented and selective law responses towards these law-breaking behaviors, as a prelude to examining the social and political environment that gave rise to the people's mediation institutions. Chapter 4 focused on the persuasion strategies in the mediation, including the mediators' characteristics, what they say, and how the strategies of the two disputing parties jointly shape the mediation outcomes from the social power perspective. Chapter 5 examines how the mediation committees applied economic compensation distribution as a solution to medical disputes and achieved the social stability maintenance goals. It also proposed the framework to understand the compensation distribution rationale in medical dispute resolution.

References

Boix, C., & Svolik, M. W. (2013) The foundations of limited authoritarian government: Institutions, commitment, and power-sharing in dictatorships. *The Journal of Politics*, 75(2): 300–316.
Cai, Y. (2008) Power structure and regime resilience: contentious politics in China. *British Journal of Political Science*, *38*(3): 411-432.
Cai Jianwen (2000) "Renmin guandian—guanyu yiliaoshigu de baogao" ("Life matters: Medical malpractice report") The North Literature and Arts Publishing House).
Chen, Z. (2009) Launch of the health-care reform plan in China. *The Lancet, 373*(9672), 1322–1324.
Chen, X. (2009) The power of "troublemaking": protest tactics and their efficacy in China. *Comparative Politics*, *41*(4): 451–471.
Chen, X. (2012) *Social protest and contentious authoritarianism in China*. Cambridge University Press.
Chen, X. (2017) Origins of informal coercion in China. *Politics & Society*, *45*(1): 67–89.
Chen Guoming, & Yang Dinge. (1993) "Hongze Xian 15 li yiliaojiufen fenxi" ("Analysis of 15 medical dispute casesin Hongze County") *(Chinese Rural Health Service Administration)*, (3): 12–13.
Cong, X. (2014) "Ma Xiwu's Way of Judging": Villages, the Masses and Legal Construction in Revolutionary China in the 1940s. *The China Journal*(72): 29–52.
Du Zhichun (2015) "Zhongguo shehui gong anquan yanjiu baogao" (Report on Chinese social public security research), (Central Compilation & Translation Press).
Eggleston, K., Ling, L., Qingyue, M., Lindelow, M., & Wagstaff, A. (2008) Health service delivery in China: a literature review. *Health economics, 17*(2): 149–165.
Feng, Y., & Zeng, Y. (2022) Stability justice: Petitioners versus non-petitioners in China's criminal adjudication. *Law & Society Review*, *56*(4): 555–579.
Fu, D. (2017a) Fragmented control: Governing contentious labor organizations in China. *Governance*, *30*(3): 445–462.
Fu, D. (2017b) Disguised collective action in China. *Comparative Political Studies*, *50*(4): 499–527.
Gallagher, M. E. (2006) Mobilizing the law in China:"Informed disenchantment" and the development of legal consciousness. *Law & Society Review*, *40*(4): 783–816.
Gandhi, J., & Przeworski, A. (2007) Authoritarian institutions and the survival of autocrats. *Comparative political studies*, *40*(11), 1279–1301.
Genschel, P. (1997) The dynamics of inertia: institutional persistence and change in telecommunications and health care. *Governance*, *10*(1): 43–66.

Huang, P. C. (2008) Centralized minimalism: Semiformal governance by quasi officials and dispute resolution in China. *Modern China, 34*(1): 9–35.
He, X. (2009) Court finance and court responses to judicial reforms: a tale of two Chinese courts. *Law & Policy, 31*(4): 463–486.
He, X. (2021) Divorce in China. In *Divorce in China.* New York University Press.
Hildebrandt, T. (2013) *Social organizations and the authoritarian state in China.* Cambridge University Press.
Hsiao, W. C. (1995) The Chinese health care system: lessons for other nations. *Social science & medicine, 41*(8): 1047–1055.
Hu, J. (2011) Grand mediation in China. *Asian Survey, 51*(6): 1065–1089.
Hu, J., & Wu, Y. (2023) Source Governance of Social Disputes in China. *Critical Asian Studies*: 1–23.
Hurst, W., & O'Brien, K. J. (2002) China's contentious pensioners. *The China Quarterly, 170*: 345–360.
Hyman, C. S., Liebman, C. B., Schechter, C. B., & Sage, W. M. (2010) Interest-based mediation of medical malpractice lawsuits: a route to improved patient safety? *Journal of health politics, policy and law, 35*(5): 797–828.
Ji Weidong. (1989) "Falv yu tiaojie de beilun " ("Repellence between Mediation and Rule of Law") (Legal Studies), (5): 21–25.
Lam, T. P., Wan, X. H., & Ip, M. S. M. (2006) Current perspectives on medical education in China. *Medical Education, 40*(10): 940–949.
Li Peilei, & Deng Yong. (2015) "Yiliao Jiufen 'xian'e siliao' tiaokuan pingjia ji gaijin jianyi" ("Policy Evaluation and Recommendation on the "pricing limit for the private negotation" in medical dispute resolution") *(Chinese Health Policy Research), 8*(9), 45–52.
Liebman, C. B., & Hyman, C. S. (2004) A mediation skills model to manage disclosure of errors and adverse events to patients. *Health Affairs, 23*(4): 22–32.
Liebman, B. L. (2013) Malpractice mobs: medical dispute resolution in China. *Columbia Law Review*: 181–264.
Mertha, A. C. (2005) China's "soft" centralization: shifting tiao/kuai authority relations. *The China Quarterly, 184*: 791–810.
Michelson, E. (2007) Climbing the dispute pagoda: grievances and appeals to the official justice system in rural China. *American sociological review, 72*(3): 459–485.
O'Brien, K. J., & Li, L. (2006) *Rightful resistance in rural China*: Cambridge University Press.
O'Brien, K. J. (1996) Rightful resistance. *World Politics, 49*(1): 31–55.
Peerenboom, R., & He, X. (2009) Dispute resolution in China: patterns, causes and prognosis. *E. Asia L. Rev., 4*, 1.
Pepinsky, T. (2014) The institutional turn in comparative authoritarianism. *British Journal of Political Science, 44*(3): 631–653.
Perry, E. J. (2008) Chinese conceptions of "rights": From Mencius to Mao—and now. *Perspectives on Politics, 6*(1): 37–50.
Qiaoan, R. (2020) State–society relations under a new model of control in China: Graduated control 2.0. *China Information, 34*(1): 24–44.
Qiu Renzong (1996) "Bingren de quanli" ("The rights of patients") (Beijing Medical University and Union Medical College of China Press).
Slater, D. (2003) Iron cage in an iron fist: Authoritarian institutions and the personalization of power in Malaysia. *Comparative Politics*: 81–101.
Studdert, D. M., Mello, M. M., Gawande, A. A., Gandhi, T. K., Kachalia, A., Yoon, C., ... & Brennan, T. A. (2006) Claims, errors, and compensation payments in medical malpractice litigation. *New England journal of medicine, 354*(19): 2024–2033.
Sun Jianguo, Mao Ronghua, Zhao Minghua (2010) "Pingheng yihuan shuangfangliyi tuoshan chuli yiliaojiufen" ("Balancing the interests of both doctors and patients and handling medical disputes properly") (People's Court Daily) (January 14, 2010), http://rmfyb.chinacourt.org/paper/images/2010-01/14/08/2010011408_pdf.pdf.

Svolik, M. (2008) Authoritarian reversals and democratic consolidation. *American Political Science Review, 102*(2): 153–168.

Tena-Tamayo, C., & Sotelo, J. (2005) Malpractice in Mexico: arbitration not litigation. *BMJ: British Medical Journal, 331*(7514): 448.

Tong, Z. (2011) "Cong 'Zhizizhishou' kan faxue rensheng: ji wujialin tang cuifang jiaoshou" (The legal life of Professor Wu Jialin and Tang Cuifang), (Social Science Forum)(6): 127–141.

Wang, J. (2015) Managing social stability: The perspective of a local government in China. *Journal of East Asian Studies, 15*(1): 1–25.

Wang, Z., & Oliphant, K. (2012) Yangge dance: the rhythm of liability for medical malpractice in the People's Republic of China. Chi.-Kent L. Rev., 87, 21.

Wang Jing. (1985) "renmin tiaojie zai zhongguo de yanxu he fazhan" (The continuity and development of people's mediation in China) (Legal Studies), *6*.

Wang Kairong. (1999) "Yiliao jiufen chuli Zhong de weishengjingji wenti" ("The health economic issues of medical dispute resolution") (Chinese Health Economics), (1): 44–45.

Wang, Y., & Minzner, C. (2015) The rise of the Chinese security state. *The China Quarterly, 222*: 339–359.

Xiaobei (1998). "Yiliao shigu heshi neng taohuige shuofa" ("How can I find justice in medical dispute resolution"), (Chinese journal of healthcare nutrition)(8): 9–11.

Xiong Yihan. (2006) "Renmin tiaojie de shehuihua yu zaizhizu:dui shanghaishi yangboshou gongzuoshi de gean fenxi" ("Socialization and re-organization of the People's Mediation: Case study of the Yang Shoubo office in Shanghai") (Sociology), *26*(6): 95–95.

Yan, X. (2016) Patrolling harmony: pre-emptive authoritarianism and the preservation of stability in W county. *Journal of Contemporary China, 25*(99), 406–421.

Yang Lixin(2003) "Minshi qinquan shizongan" ("Ten cases of civil infringement")方圆 (Fangyuan)7.

Yee, F. (2005) Mandatory Mediation: The Extra Dose Needed to Cure the Medical Malpractice Crisis. *Cardozo J. Conflict Resol., 7*, 393.

Zhou, L. (2023) Mediation and grassroots policing in China: Conflict resolution or social control?. *China Information, 37*(2): 165–184.

Zhuang, W., & Chen, F. (2015) "Mediate First": The revival of mediation in labour dispute resolution in China. *The China Quarterly, 222*: 380–402.

Chapter 3
Understanding Hospital Violence in China

> 无偷赏，无赦罚
> Never reward and punish arbitrarily.
> ——韩非子《主道》in Han Feizi [The way of the ruler]
> 不赦死，不宥刑，赦死宥刑，是谓威淫。
> Do not pardon capital crimes or reduce punishment; otherwise, the country will be in danger, and the power of the country will fall by the wayside.
> ——韩非子《爱臣》in Han Feizi [Favored Ministers]

This chapter examines extreme medical disputes—hospital violence—and the government's responses. In the first decade of the 2000s, violence against doctors (*yinao*) in the workplace was repeatedly reported. As a new type of social conflict, hospital violence is easily and quickly politicized and escalates into mass incidents targeting health institutions. This chapter aims to fill the scholarly gap in tracing the government responses towards hospital violence and its outcomes. I first theorize the behaviors of hospital violence from the rightful resistance perspective by examining their mobilizing structure, framing strategies, sequential targeting tactics, etc. Drawing on intensive interviews and media data, I find that the government has adopted selective punishment to avoid blame and dispute escalation. This chapter demonstrates that the government's selective punishment strategies are contingent upon three factors: (1) the degree of violence, (2) the disputants' strategies, and (3) the disputants' moral power. This study suggests that selective law enforcement has led hospitals to adopt self-protection strategies and has provided further political space for disruptive behaviors in health institutions.

3.1 From "Empty Nose Syndrome" to Hospital Violence

Empty nose syndrome (ENS, *kongbi zheng*, 空鼻症) is a rare disorder without a clear definition and treatment. According to a nascent medical study, ENS is an iatrogenic disorder most often recognized for the presence of paradoxical nasal obstruction after the widely performed patent nasal fossa. Patients with ENS have commonly

J. Wu, *Politicized Medical Dispute Resolution in China*, Understanding China,
https://doi.org/10.1007/978-981-97-6961-2_3

experienced anxiety and depression disorder, as they often relate it to a sense of suffocation (Chhabra & Houser, 2009) and complain that each breath hurts like a knife cut.[1] However, this rare condition is well known to medical workers in China because it has led to several cases of violence in Chinese hospitals.

In China, patients with ENS have been involved in violent incidents, attacking doctors in public hospitals. For instance, on 25 October 2013, a patient named Lian Enqing连恩清 attacked three doctors in the outpatient department of a public hospital in Wenling 温岭 (a district in Zhejiang Province), killing one and stabbing two others before being overpowered by a security guard.[2] The following day, nearly one hundred doctors and nurses wearing masks and white coats assembled in the square of the Wenling People's Hospital, carrying banners expressing their sorrow over the death of Doctor Wang Yunjie (王云杰) and asking for dignity and safety in the workplace. The public petition also won the online support of workers in hundreds of hospitals nationwide.[3]

However, there is also the patient's side to the story. Patient Lian was a pitiable man whose pain no one understood. There was no official name for his symptoms at that time. After nasal surgery, his situation worsened, and he could not breathe normally. Even his family members did not understand his torment, assuming he just felt dry in his nose, which they dismissed as not a big deal. In reality, every breath devastated the poor man, who was no longer the man he used to be. For years, Lian could neither sleep nor work, causing his family economic hardship. In August 2013, he was sent to a mental hospital, where he was diagnosed as having long-term psychological depression. Ten days after his release, he targeted the doctors he blamed for his "unsatisfactory" treatments and committed his violent crime, leading to one causality and two injuries.[4] Neither during his trial, nor while in prison, nor during a TV interview did he show remorse for his crime, instead insisting that the doctor had "asked for it."[5]

Lian's case is not unique. In Beijing, Mr. Wang, a well-known artist who specialized in painting, brutally stabbed his surgeon,[6] whom he blamed for ruining his life by

---

[1] Fieldwork in C city in August 2017, as well as see, "Empty nose syndrome" group: The air I breathe in is like a knife, http://news.sohu.com/20161130/n474490236.shtml, accessed on September 19, 2023.

[2] See, for instance, The defendant in the "October 25" doctor-killing case in Wenling, Zhejiang Province was sentenced to death in the first instance, https://www.gov.cn/jrzg/2014-01/27/content_2576849.htm, accessed on September 19, 2023.

[3] See, for instance,The doctor-killing case in Wenling, https://news.ifeng.com/opinion/special/wenlingshayi/, accessed on September 19, 2023.

[4] See, for instance, [No. 1286] Lian Enqing intentional homicide case—How to combine clinical diagnosis and judicial psychiatric evaluation opinions to accurately determine the defendant's criminal responsibility at the time of the crime? http://www.drxsfd.com/xf/anli.asp?bh=3524, accessed on September 19, 2023.

[5] See, for instance, Lian Enqing, the murderer who killed a doctor in Wenling, Zhejiang: Doctors deserve to be punished for their own actions, https://www.guancha.cn/local/2014_04_07_220138.shtml, accessed on October 25, 2023.

[6] See, for instance, The cost of blood: Case of hospital violence in Tongren, http://www.infzm.com/content/63318, accessed on Dec 7, 2016.

performing nasal surgery. Wang expressed no regret and received the death penalty due to the severe damage he caused.

Doctors in other ENT (Ear, Nose and Throat) departments have also been violently attacked by patients, including Doctor Dai Wenhong (killed in Henan province in 2007), Doctor Sun Dongtao (killed in Beigang hospital in 2015), and Doctor Xu Wen (who suffered a chopping wound in Tongren Hospital in Beijing in 2011). These attacks drew widespread attention to safety in hospitals. Commenting on the repeated violent incidents in hospitals, Doctor Wu, who practiced in the ENT department of a famous hospital, complained:

> Now, I am very cautious in dealing with nasal operations. My team and I check and make phone calls to every patient after they receive treatment to ensure they are doing fine. You know, I cannot risk my life and my family's happiness. We need to protect ourselves.[7]

Conflicts with doctors quickly escalate into discontent with public institutions, and perpetrators win public support due to media exposure. Incidents of hospital violence feature high mobilization power: the size and organizational abilities of these conflicts could expand rapidly, threatening the stability of public institutions and even society. The linkages between heightened action and disruptive actions are often short. Although the government prioritizes dealing with regime-threatening conflicts and social disputes to maintain social order and stability, hospital violence has become a new category of mass incidents that must be reported annually (Du, 2015).

In addition to the extremely violent crimes discussed above, hospital violence takes many other forms. In China, more than half of medical practitioners reported having experienced repeated verbal or physical violence in the workplace (Fang, 2015). Violence in hospitals (*yinao*) endangers professionals' workplace security and severely violates the law, threatening grassroots social stability and rule-of-law governance. Repeated incidents of hospital violence (*yinao*) in recent years have prompted the government to pay attention to maintaining social order in hospitals.

Extant explanations of hospital violence have focused on the effect of patient-doctor distrust, a problematic health system, and economic perspectives. For instance, medical studies often attribute hospital violence to the privatization of China's health system, unqualified health treatment, and low health insurance reimbursement rates, which have led to doctor-patient distrust (Tucker et al., 2015; Milcent, 2016). However, few studies have examined the political and legal responses to such violence (an exception being Huang, 2021). The Chinese government has long attached great importance and efforts to stability maintenance to prevent social and political disturbances. Hospital violence is also a form of resistance openly displayed on the street that could translate into mobilization and organization capacity, attracting government intervention.

To fill this gap, this chapter studies hospital violence from a political perspective, asking what political space hospital violence possesses and how the government

[7] Interview with a doctor on March 2016 from the ENT department in a tertiary hospital in the C city.

and hospitals deal with it. It examines hospital violence through the lens of rightful resistance and compares 155 cases of hospital violence (collected from various media channels) to explore the government's flexible strategies for dealing with it. The cases had varying characteristics, including different tactics, modes of violence, degree of violence, and resultant penalties. From 2015 to 2017, I visited some of the involved hospitals and local juridical bureaus in various districts several times to communicate with doctors, juridical and police officials and study front-line workers' varied strategies for dealing with this violence.

This chapter first categorizes and theoretically defines the concept of hospital violence using social movement theories. Then, it examines the government's dynamic strategies in dealing with hospital violence and compares various sanctions and punishments associated with hospital violence cases. Maintaining social stability and being responsive to citizens' grievances is a daily dilemma local officials face when upholding the law. Although the government has criminalized disrupting hospitals' daily operations, rule-breakers often receive tolerant or lenient treatment.

This chapter contributes to the literature on contentious politics and the rule of law in several ways. First, it provides empirical evidence by analyzing different modes of hospital violence from a political participation perspective. Primarily drawing upon media reports, fieldwork and interviews, it studies how patients adopt various resistance tactics to reflect their perceptions of justice and protect rights. Second, it observes street-level law enforcement officials' selective punishment style when coping with hospital violence. In China, local officials refrain from coercive repression, instead substituting selective punishment to cope with bottom-up personal grievances and avoid blame. The nature of hospital violence, the degree of violence, and patients' moral power jointly shape the government's perception of risks and flexible response strategies. By analyzing the government's rationale for selective punishment, this chapter also contributes to understanding China's fragmented social stability maintenance system, which provides the background for revitalizing people's mediation.

3.2 Methods

The empirical evidence of this chapter is based on media reports and an intensive fieldwork investigation of the daily practices of law enforcement among local officials. From 2015 to 2017, I collected 155 cases of hospital violence from 2010 to 2017 from the China Digital Library database and conducted face-to-face interviews with medical workers, police, and juridical workers (see Appendix for details). I used the keywords "hospital violence" (*yinao* 医闹) and "violence against doctor" (*shangyi* 伤医) to collect the cases. The descriptive data for each case of hospital violence include the type of citizen, date, hospital name, hospital level, number of participants, whether a patient's death was involved, whether casualty or severe injury resulted, and punishment received. The cases cover 22 provinces, with three places—Guangdong, Shanghai, and Hunan—having the most frequent incidents of

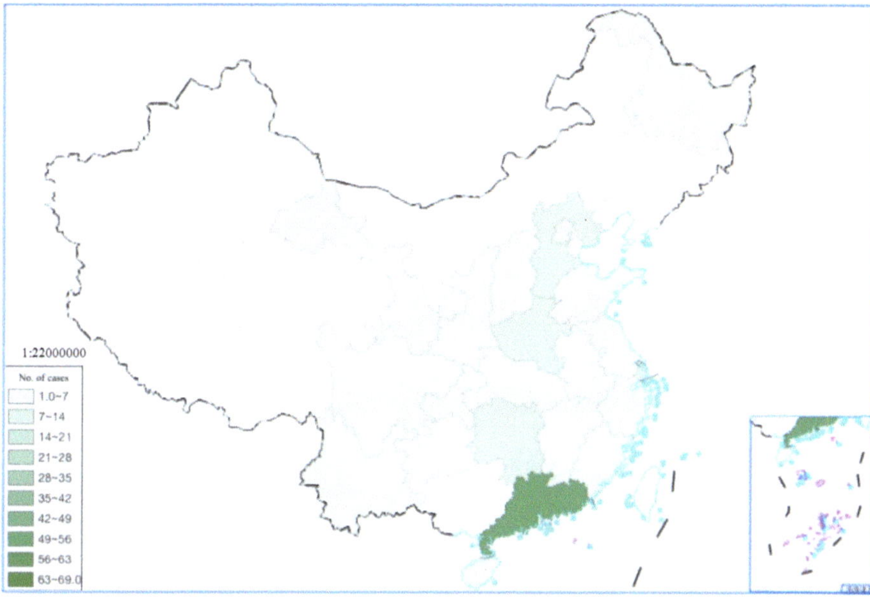

Fig. 3.1 Geographic distribution of cases of hospital violence

hospital violence. Despite some inherent biases and the small sample size, the data are valuable for examining cases of hospital violence and the government's coping strategy (Fig. 3.1).

The reasons for hospital violence varied greatly. Drawing upon empirical evidence from government reports and internal hospital documents, the most frequent reasons (the death of a patient, discontent with treatment results, and long wait times) accounted for approximately 80% of all hospital violence. Other causes include the effects of alcohol, mental disorders, economic compensation claims, etc. In addition, to better observe the government's mindset and coping strategy, I interviewed front-line hospital workers, juridical officials, and police officers dealing with hospital violence cases. I contacted five interviewees through personal connections and the remainder through the snowball approach. Most respondents held middle to senior positions in a public hospital or local authority investigating incidents of hospital violence; all were front-line workers with at least seven years of experience addressing hospital violence. Specifically, the respondents were asked, "What is your/your hospital's procedure for addressing hospital violence?" (Fig. 3.2).

The associated punishments patients received were traced through: (1) trial results in the Court Verdict Web of the Supreme People's Court of PRC, (2) follow-up news on *Dingxiang Web* (an online web alliance of healthcare professionals), and (3) public notices published by hospitals. Despite progress in developing China's stability maintenance institutions, fewer than half of hospital violence cases resulted in penalties. When conducting the fieldwork, I frequently heard complaints from medical workers that local officials had weak capabilities and low motivation to

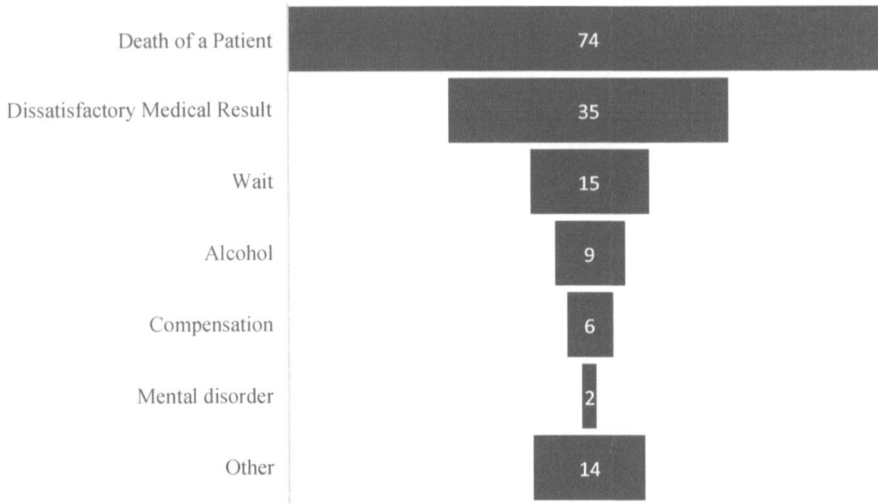

Fig. 3.2 Causes of hospital violence. *Source* Author's database

address hospital violence, and not all patients or their family members who committed hospital violence were punished. In the findings, I combine content analysis and fieldwork to explain the logic of the punishment mechanism for hospital violence in China by categorizing various levels and punishments and the characteristics of the associated disruptive acts.

The following section first defines hospital violence from a political perspective and examines how citizens utilize it to protect their rights and hold hospitals and the government accountable. Next, it traces the government's inconsistent and selective punishment towards hospital violence. Despite disruptive actions in hospitals being criminalized, local officials often constrained their use of coercion and sanctions to avoid being blamed by the public or intensifying the conflict. Selective punishment also reflected the government's dilemma in maintaining grassroots social order. In other words, the government's hands were tied, limiting its institutional responses to medical disputes.

3.3 Hospital Violence as a Form of Resistance

From a political perspective, I define hospital violence as a form of resistance applied by aggrieved citizens to address medical disputes. Since China's reform and opening up in the late 1970s, citizens have increasingly adopted rightful resistance as a form of political participation to proactively protect their rights. Likewise, the organizational tactics of hospital violence resemble those of other acts of popular resistance in China in many ways. For instance, some patients have applied non-violent strategies (*wennao*, 文闹), such as verbal threats and insults or displaying coffins in public spaces, with a lower degree of law-breaking. Others have resorted to physical violence (*wunao*, 武闹), including attacking doctors and nurses, kidnapping medical professionals and their family members, or forcing them to kneel in public. Patients have shown high internal solidarity and rapid mobilization capacity in holding hospitals accountable. Hospital violence overtly expresses anger and a political intention to hold public institutions accountable and ensure they prioritize patients' demands in addressing grievances. Although the disputes occur in hospitals, citizens could quickly shift their target to the local government to hold it accountable. This form of resistance does not necessarily challenge regime legitimacy but aims to attract local officials' attention and accelerate the problem-addressing process as the "weapon of the weak" (Scott, 1985). Hence, cases of *yinao* used to be handled and intervened in through local governments' micro-management and direct intervention (Liu et al., 2020; Huang, 2021), rather than legal channels. This section first analyses hospital violence from the perspective of rightful resistance by examining its mobilizing structure, how grievances are presented, and sequential targeting, key elements of hospital violence.

It is worth noting that hospital violence is not synonymous with medical disputes. Though some hospital violence derives from medical disputes, it is law-breaking behavior that sometimes results in death or injuries to innocent citizens. From the government's perspective, hospital violence contains higher risks and threatens the safety of citizens and health institutions. Observing dynamic government responses to these law-breaking behaviors would help examine government strategies for stability maintenance and the rule of law in China.

3.3.1 Mobilizing Structure

The mobilization structure of hospital violence is worth noting, as it shapes various local government responses. Many scholars have acknowledged the crucial role of social networks in mobilizing social movements (see, for instance, Snow et al., 1980; Gould, 1991; Parkinson, 2013), yet few have compared the efficacy of various types of mobilization structures and how governments perceive their level of risk, let alone differentiated the mobilizing structure in hospital violence scenarios.

Drawing from the fieldwork and casefile, I categorize the mobilization structure of hospital violence into three types, based on (1) social ties, such as close family members, clans, friends etc., (2) economic ties that mainly pursue materialist interests; and (3) moral ties usually driven by altruism, sympathy, voluntariness, etc.[8] Different mobilization structures predict various degrees of "moral legitimacy" related to cultural norms, shaping various government coping strategies.

---

[8] In reality, one incident of hospital violence may combine various types of social ties.

First, the mobilization through social ties model refers to a process in which hospital violence is organized and participated in by patients' family members, friends, or clans whose close-knit social ties could generate shared grievances. In the model, actors' linkages between heightened emotion and disruptive behaviors are short, and their natural kin-based social relations could rapidly translate into mobilization power and a propensity for collective actions. For instance, in the Nanping case in Fujian Province (discussed in Chapter Two), shared grief over the death of a clan member mobilized Yang villagers to undertake large-scale collective actions in the hospital.

A similar case also occurred in the fieldwork city in 2011. Mr. L, a non-local patient from A City, traveled with his son to C City under doctors' advice to undergo surgery. However, Mr. L later died from a post-surgery infection, costing the family 300 thousand RMB—an unaffordable economic burden that forced the L family to sell their house. After Mr. L's death, his family protested what they saw as useless treatments, and six family members, including his son, daughter, sister, and brother-in-law, surrounded the doctor's office to resolve their medical dispute. However, the doctor's "indifferent" attitude unexpectedly led to a group fight at the hospital. The deceased patient's son stabbed the doctor and was detained by the police, while others received warnings or administrative penalties. According to the son, he just wanted "an explanation from the doctors," but the hospital representative refused to speak with them. One juridical official I interviewed recalled this incident and showed great sympathy towards the patients, saying, "the patient's family members were waiting for medical dispute mediation in the office. However, the tragedy happened before the police officers could arrive, and everyone lost control."[9] He is not alone; when facing criticism from the hospital, police from the public security bureau described the patient family as coming from "disadvantaged groups" (*ruoshiqunti* 弱势群体), commenting that.

> They were just regular people (not organized hospital mobs), and we could feel their pain. We (police officers) communicated with them before the tragedy occurred and persuaded them to seek help through institutional channels (e.g., the courts). But they seemed to have limited knowledge of how to protect their right appropriately and said they acted out of 'filial piety'孝.[10]

The social tie-based mobilization structure presents high mobilizing capacity but entails high moral power. The hospital criticized the "sympathy" shown to the family by the police, juridical officers, and the public. On 9 February 2011, one doctor wrote, in an online BBS, that "(T)he weather is so cold outside, but not comparable to my heart.... As long as the government does not promulgate measures to protect the rights of doctors, the media's unilateral and biased reports will lead to more such violence against doctors."[11] As society prioritizes filial piety, the public often demonstrates high sympathy for grieving patients' and their families. To some extent, their aggrieved behaviors do not "deviate from culturally accepted levels of dissent,"

[9] Interview with a juridical worker involved in August 2016.

[10] Interview with one local official in August 2016.

[11] Author's archived data.

using Davenport's term (1995), and are often compatible with the traditional culture in the target society. Hence, the government will allow or "acquiesce" to these types of disruptive actions, rather than resort to direct repression.

In comparison, the economic ties model refers to protesters engaging in hospital violence for material gain but not sharing social connections with the patients. According to Liebman (2013), professional "malpractice mobs," lured by potential economic returns, pressure hospital representatives by staging disruptive actions to extort high monetary compensation. These hospital mobs do not share close natural ties with the patient but instrumentally rally in exchange for economic gain. According to a media survey, professional hospital mobs often have a pyramidal division of labor.[12] Senior and middle-aged women are paid 300 RMB per day to participate in non-violent activities, such as entranceway sit-ins, to attract public attention, while young males (often disguised as relatives of the patient) verbally threaten doctors and nurses for 500 RMB a day. Payments are much higher if the patient requests that their doctor be beaten and could include funds to hire a professional lawyer.

Hospital mobs do not often resort to violent behaviors; instead, aware of the boundaries of the law, they often use disruptive but non-violent approaches like raising banners and crying in public spaces to attract bystanders' attention and leverage their bargaining power in negotiating with hospitals. Their goal is to lessen the "face" of the hospitals, which they believe could accelerate the dispute-solving process. One hospital mob leader stated, "The utmost rule is that you could watch from the outside, and make noise, but you must not use your fists."[13] The ultimate goal of the hospital mob is to embarrass and place psychological pressure on hospitals rather than pursue "eye-for-eye" justice, as they are well aware of the political cost of exerting violence against doctors directly. Monetary pursuits are often their primary objectives. After initiating a disruptive action, the lead of the hospital mob would bargain with the hospital for more compensation, while the hospital mobs would receive no less than an eight percent commission.[14] When examining government strategies, it is important to distinguish between mobilization structures based on social and economic ties, as the latter often result in sanctions. The occurrence and proliferation of professional mobs have demoralized and delegitimated patients' claims, and local officials are more likely to apply repression or legal weapons to penalize them.

Third, a less likely scenario concerns the actions of bystanders or conscious participants in hospital violence based on moral ties—i.e., allies motivated by social conscience or moral outrage, empathy, anger, or misinformation (Habermas, 1990; Van Stekelenburg, 2013; Van Stekelenburg et al., 2009; Duncan, 1999; Wahlström,

[12] See, for instance, Exploring the secrets of professional medical troublemakers: 100 yuan per person per day, 20% of the profit if successful, https://www.chinanews.com.cn/fz/2013/11-21/5531557.shtml, accessed on September 20, 2023.

[13] See, for instance, A big reveal of professional "medical troublemakers": blackmailing the hospital and then extorting the family members, http://hunan.voc.com.cn/article/201407/201407010756374425.html, accessed on September 20, 2023.

[14] Ibid.

Peterson, & Wennerhag, 2018) who participated in the collective action spontaneously and voluntarily, without thought of receiving direct material benefits. Typical examples are White people at Black Lives Matter protests (e.g., Luttrell, 2019) and White students from elite families engaging in civil rights movements (e.g., Wiles, 2001). When pre-existing ties are absent, moral shock can become a source of strangers' involvement (Jasper & Poulsen, 1995). Mobilization structures based on moral ties are the most likely to escalate into mass incidents and, though rare, attract the most government attention.

Hospital violence that attracts many bystanders shows a high degree of spontaneity without organization and threatens social stability, but only occurs under certain circumstances. For example, in 2012, a female non-local resident received an IV treatment in a hospital in Dongguan, Guangdong Province, and died the next morning.[15] At first, a dozen of the woman's relatives surrounded and created a disturbance at the hospital. However, the number of participants unexpectedly grew to nearly 2000 the next day, creating what could be the largest incidence of hospital violence in China. Most protestors were "conscience adherents" (McCarthy and Zald, 1977) motivated by their empathy for non-local or vulnerable persons subjected to injustice or careless treatment. The Dongguan City local government had to dispatch large numbers of police to disperse participants and discourage a mass incident.

Collective actions based on moral ties are highly likely to transform medical disputes into mass incidents by resonating with the public's empathy over unjust situations. A similar case occurred in Shanghai, where, after a migrant worker's pregnant wife miscarried, a sense of shared grievance, sympathy, anger, and dissatisfaction mobilized many migrant workers to surround the hospital. The incorporation of conscience adherents based on moral ties fueled and sustained the collective action. Conscience participants' mobilizing structure can be based on shared acquaintance, similar experiences of grievance or discrimination, general principles of justice, unexamined rumors, etc., and can be a nightmare for local officials. Therefore, the government has made great efforts to prevent the emergence of conscience participants and organizations based on moral ties.

3.3.2 *Sequential Targeting*

Although the primary target of patients' resistance is the hospital believed to be directly responsible for their grievances, it has been widely observed that patients often shift their focus to local government to hold it accountable, accelerate the dispute resolution process, and prioritize their demands. According to Chen and Cai (2021), ordinary Chinese protestors readily differentiate between "whom to blame" and "whom to ask for help" (p. 3), leading to "upward targeting behaviors" in collective actions to hold higher-level government departments accountable. In addressing medical disputes, patients do not turn to local health bureaus for help; instead, they

[15] Author's own database.

frequently target local government to change the status quo, as it is believed to have more political importance and greater capacity to dispense justice. In comparison, the dubious father-son relations between hospitals and supervisory health bureaus prevent citizens' reliance on the latter.

Patients' common targeting sequence is to hold the involved doctors and nurses responsible; however, patients believe their vulnerability, underprivileged status, and information asymmetry prevent them from getting the truth from hospitals and healthcare professionals directly. Next, they escalate their target, turning to the local government for help punishing the "wrongdoers," believing it has more capacity to influence health institutions. If the local government fails to be responsive, increased disruptions or even petitions to higher-level government may ensue. The escalation and target shifting signal an escalation to collective action featuring evolving and more disruptive tactics. In China, the government has become the favored target of protesters seeking help, regardless of the nature of the conflict. For instance, workers from private enterprises often petition local governments for unpaid wages in labour disputes, as governments are considered omnipotent and responsible for all social conflicts (Chen, 2003). If the local government fails to address these social disputes, whether through perceived misconduct, inaction, or dubious interlocked interests with hospitals, protestors shift the focus of their anger, targeting higher-level government or even the political system writ large, upgrading their modes of political participation, an outcome local governments want most to prevent.

Though local governments are not directly involved in medical disputes, patients still hold them accountable and consider them crucial actors in making the final call or intervening to balance the scales. Therefore, local governments face the dilemma of deciding whether to accommodate patients' claims. On the one hand, failing to address patients' grievances may shift the protestors' focus to higher government. Patients often blame local governments for their inaction, suspecting them of planning to help hospitals cover up their wrongdoings. Some even leverage their influence through upward petitioning, which often signals the local government's weakness and incompetence. For instance, in a famous 2010 case in Yongzhou, Hunan Province,[16] Patient T complained that the hospital failed to detect her ectopic pregnancy symptoms, leading to the loss of her right fallopian tube. According to the hospital, Patient T "harassed" the hospital for two years, threatening it and local officials many times that she would petition Beijing. Patient T, however, claimed she had visited Beijing to meet with lawyers and journalists rather than to petition higher government. Under the pressure of skip-level petitioning, the involved hospital agreed to provide 60,000 RMB in compensation, transferred indirectly via the local government's poverty alleviation fund.[17] Under the "stability at all costs" mindset, the local government was motivated to satisfy the patient's claims to avoid her petitioning behaviors.

On the other hand, accommodating patients' claims at all costs inevitably encourages other patients to replicate such targeting practices, to the hospitals' detriment. In extreme cases, governments' over-tolerance could backfire, mobilizing medical

[16] Author's own database.

[17] The patient was later detained for "picking quarrels and provoking troubles".

workers to protect their rights through collective actions. For instance, in December 2015 in Yongqing County, Hebei Province, a deceased patient's family forced three doctors to kneel before the corpse, stabbing one of them. Police at the scene did not offer immediate help, saying they "had not received orders."[18] The next morning, nearly one hundred doctors and nurses took to the streets with banners stating, "It is a violation of law to detain [doctors]," and petitioned the local government to express their discontent. A similar case occurred in Nanping, Fujian Province, after the local government reached a private agreement with patients without a full investigation. Lavish and repeated overcompensation of patients has reduced healthcare professionals' authority and increased hospitals' financial burdens (Li & Deng, 2015).

Patients' sequential targeting strategy has politicized the nature of medical disputes. Local governments make constant trade-offs between hospitals and patients based on either side's potential political threat or resistance level. From local officials' perspectives, closing disputes efficiently before protesters shift their target to local government is the wisest course of action.

3.3.3 *Make a Scene: Open Art of Resistance*

A "scene" is a kind of place, having both a material (location) and a mental (cultural or symbolic) meaning. As suggested by Goffman's (2017) face-to-face interactions theory, to challenge authority one could make a scene, an open act of resistance. In cases of hospital violence, protesters often increase their bargaining power in negotiating with hospitals and local government by making a confrontational, unpleasant, and dramatic scene to forestall repression or sanctions by publicly displaying their grievances, desperation, and outrage to arouse empathy and affection. It is often adopted as the power of the weak, such as in the gay rights movements of the mid-1960s and the more recent "Me-Too" protests, whose participants carried a 50-pound mattress around campus (McDonald, 2019), collectively developing and fostering a culture scene. As Blom and Jaoul (2008) noted, the use of moral and emotional claims that resonate with the target cultural environment is always innovative and persuasive. This is also true in China's context.

Displaying a coffin in a public space has become common in hospital violence cases, aiming to attract sympathy from conscious bystanders and local officials, increase protester's moral power, and arouse the public's moral indignation. For instance, in Hainan (case no. 148), a child's death agitated their whole family,[19] who convened 300 villagers to place the child's coffin in the hospital's lobby. As a part of the demonstration, the family created a banner stating, "Medical Disputes, Pay with Your Life." Officials have often have shown great compassion in dealing with such unpleasant scenes, despite the large number of protesters involved. Local

[18] Author's own database.

[19] Based on author's database.

police intervened but only arrested eight leading participants, freeing the rest. The eight leaders received an administrative penalty and were released 15 days later.

The scenes created by protesters defy widely acknowledged social and cultural norms in the target society. In Chinese culture, displaying the deceased's coffin or body conveys the symbolic cultural meaning of "grievances" (*yuan* 冤), demands that one show respect to the deceased. Dating back to the Tsing dynasty, moving or exposing a coffin would result in legal penalties, as a show of respect for the deceased and their families and bureaucratic efforts to regulate the body (Snyder-Reinke, 2016). Today, protestors often force hospital representatives or involved doctors to bow to or even kneel before coffins placed in hospital lobbies. While front-line police are aware that such scenes violate public security administration and punishment regulations, the embedded cultural meaning ties their hands and they cannot resort to repression. One police officer explained his considerations when dealing with such cases:

> I was called to the hospital and found the family had placed the body of the deceased child, joss money, sticks and candles, which jammed the hospital's lobby and scared many patients away. The hospital was afraid to irritate the parents and took no further action. I talked to the parents directly and showed remorse for their boy. I told them to remove the coffin from the hospital lobby to help the little boy find some peace, while permitting them to keep some flowers and lit candles as a concession. Using force in these cases is risky as it could easily lead to escalation; such flexibility is often very common in our daily exercising of law.[20]

Because there is a lack of mutual trust and institutional channels to address medical disputes, citizens resort to open resistance, adopting cultural symbols relating to their cultural institutions to air their grievances. Likewise, Taiwan scholars also note that patient families display coffins in public spaces to create a sorrowful atmosphere and attract media attention, further deteriorating patient-doctor relations (Chiu, 2007). The media often publicizes scenes to attract viewers or readers. As discussed, making a scene aims to arouse the public's moral indignation and distrust in hospitals by emphasizing patients' grievances and powerlessness. It evokes bystanders', the media's, and local officials' empathy by holding them morally responsible. However, it also reproduces the power asymmetry between patients and doctors and further blurs the nature of medical disputes; identifying the causes of medical disputes and attributing responsibility are no longer priorities. Moral indignation towards doctors and hospitals may also put local government in an awkward position for failing to provide necessary assistance to patients and protect doctors.

[20] Interview with the police officer in August 2017 in C city.

3.4 Safe Hospital Project and Selective Punishment

3.4.1 Background

In 2014, President Xi Jinping delivered a speech at the Chinese People's Political Consultative Conference (CPPCC), publicly assigning blame for violence in public hospitals to restore social order. Xi stated the importance of "maintaining order in hospitals and protecting the safety of medical staff," emphasizing that "any law-breaking behaviors against doctors and nurses should be penalized seriously, in accordance with the law."[21] The then Premier of the State Council, Li Keqiang 李克强, also commented, "The relevant departments should attach great importance to this issue, and effective measures should be applied to maintain order in the medical field.[22]"

China's leadership has shown its political commitment to maintaining social order in the workplace. Under top-down pressure, legal and administrative regulations have been put in place through the Safe Hospital Project (*pingan yiyuan,* 平安医院), requiring various political authorities to address hospital violence and avoid the spread of organized social unrest. The regulations provide detailed guidance on strategies for maintaining safety and public security, including establishing and upgrading safety infrastructures and increasing security by hiring professional security guards.[23] The Safe Hospital Project tasks various institutions with maintaining social stability at hospitals, including public security bureaus, juridical authorities, insurance enterprises, hospitals, and propaganda bureaus. For example, as core stability maintenance institutions, public security bureaus focus on crime crack-downs and maintaining social order through harsh strategies. Stability maintenance system partners include juridical departments, health institutions, propaganda institutions, and other government authorities, leveraging and consolidating departmental resources to tackle problems collectively. Other new partners include semi-public agents like public institutions and state-owned enterprises. For instance, insurance companies decrease disturbances by promoting medical liability insurance as a means of risk management and conflict resolution (Luo et al., 2021). The Project reflects an "all-encompassing stability maintenance system" that includes all necessary political authorities collaborating to prevent and contain collective actions in contemporary China.

Among the new regulations, the introduction of the propaganda department is interesting. Since 2010, internal regulations collectively issued by the Ministry

---

[21] See, for instance, Xi Jinping responds to frequent medical troubles: Behavior that harms doctors must be severely punished in accordance with the law, http://npc.people.com.cn/n/2014/0308/c376899-24569312.html, accessed on September 23, 2023.

[22] See, for instance, Li Keqiang pays close attention to the Wenling doctor-killing incident and demands that medical order be maintained, http://www.chinanews.com/gn/2013/11-01/5450303.shtml, accessed on September 23, 2023.

[23] "Guidance on Strengthening the Safety Infrastructure of Hospital Safety" (Department of Public Security and National Health and Health Commission, Document No. 28, 2013).

of Justice 司法部, Ministry of Health卫生部, and China Insurance Regulatory Commission 保监会 have incorporated propaganda departments to educate the public and society and change public opinion. The policy reads,

> The whole propaganda system should focus on producing positive publicity reports, such as health practitioners' continuous efforts and sacrifices. Additionally, the propaganda should set examples for doctors with extraordinary medical skills for the public. Most importantly, the media should also increase public awareness of the limitations of the medical disciplines and encourage acceptance of the risks in the medical service.[24]

By involving propaganda institutions, the integrated social stability mechanism sought to rebuild the image of health practitioners by encouraging more positive propaganda for the healthcare system to lead and transform public opinion, addressing the root causes of hospital violence. The interviewee from the juridical authority explained,

> Actually, hospital violence is not reported as often as it was. Previously, hospital violence often attracted too much unwanted media attention. Nowadays, the regulation re-emphasizes that the role of public propaganda is to lead and guide public opinion to create a more favorable environment for doctors. We need to borrow and rely on propaganda to shape public opinion.[25]

News coverage used to highlight patients' conflicts and grievances, blurring the nature of the medical dispute to attract viewers. For instance, in 2011, a newborn baby in Shenzhen was diagnosed with Hirschsprung disease—a rare birth defect in which the child's intestines are blocked. The doctors suggested surgery estimated to cost 100,000 RMB.[26] The parents refused and sought a second opinion from another hospital, which prescribed paraffin oil, an effective treatment that cost only 0.8 RMB. The parents complained to the media and were suspicious that the first hospital sought to perform unnecessary, expensive surgery for monetary gain. The sharp contrast between 100,000 and 0.8 yuan led to public criticism of the hospital's profit-driven behaviors. One netizen commented, "It is common hospital practice to make money."[27] The widespread criticism forced the hospital to publicly state that its doctors had made a judgement call that was morally sound and technically right for the patient, clarifying that the estimated cost was 25,000 RMB, not the 100,000 RMB claimed by the parents.[28] To everyone's surprise, further medical examination

[24] Opinions on Strengthening People's Mediation of Medical Disputes" (Notice of Ministry of Justice, Ministry of Health and China Insurance Regulatory Commission, Document No. 5, 2010).

[25] Interview with the public hospital representative in C city, July 2017.

[26] According to the hospital, their estimated price was 25,000, instead to 100,000. See, for instance, Truth Investigation: Investigation of the "8 dime" Incident, http://news.cntv.cn/society/20111115/119604.shtml, accessed on September 22, 2023.

[27] See, for instance, The baby was diagnosed with a 100,000 yuan surgery, but he was cured with 80 cents of medicine, https://news.sina.com.cn/c/2011-09-08/065723124447.shtml, accessed on September 22, 2023.

[28] See, for instance, The child underwent successful surgery at Tongji Hospital, the parents wrote a letter to apologize to Shenzhen Children's Hospital, https://www.tjh.com.cn/TjhNews/20111029_11338.html, accessed on September 22, 2023.

confirmed the first doctor's diagnosis. The parents later publicly apologized to the involved doctors and hospital.

Lured by "viewer traffic," the media prefers to expose the power asymmetry between doctors and vulnerable patients and the conflictual nature of medical disputes. Media rarely investigate the facts of medical disputes, and coverage is often biased and superficial (Huang, 2021), further deteriorating patient-doctor relations. As a result, media coverage of hospital violence has decreased the number of students choosing medicine majors in college entrance exams (Bo et al., 2020). Even worse, media coverage has sometimes led to the de facto diffusion of disruptive tactics by popularizing troublemaking tactics and familiarizing patients with them. Therefore, the Safe Hospital Project incorporates the public media into the chain of command to avoid biased reports and rebuild patient-doctor trust in the health system.

A noteworthy and crucial change in the Safe Hospital Project is its revision of the Public Security Punishment Law. After Xi's speech at the People's Consultative Conference, a collective proposal initiated by 90 representatives listed health institutions as public spaces under the protection of the public security departments, revising the 23rd article of the Public Security Punishment Law. The government applied legal weapons to criminalize hospital violence, de-legitimatize disruptive tactics in hospitals, and demoralize protesters. Feng and Zeng (2022) termed the phenomenon "stability justice," which refers to the instrumental use of law and criminal procedures to deter citizens' disruptive claims while maintaining governance legitimacy and restoring social order. Penalties for disruptive actions could be fines of up to 500 RMB, five to ten days' detention, or even criminal charges.

Doctrinally, these regulations aimed to restore order in hospitals and ensure the safety of health institutions. Though considered China's harshest-ever strategy for dealing with hospital violence, few studies have examined its efficacy and de jure law enforcement in hospitals. How do front-line officials respond to hospital violence, and to what extent had the Safe Hospital Project protected and restored the social order in health institutions.

3.4.2 Selective Punishment and Its Rationale

This study empirically examines the government's responses to and punishments for hospital violence. Media case files show that street-level law enforcement has remained selective and inconsistent. Although the government has decisively condemned hospital disturbances, front-line local officials have refrained from enforcing the letter of the law. Rather than using integrated and coordinated measures to punish lawbreakers, local officials often apply selective punishment to avoid getting blamed and agitating disputants when dealing with hospital violence. Local officials enjoy discretional power when enforcing the law at the street level and can ignore popular and unmeasurable policies that conflict with their interests (Hanser, 2016; O'Brien & Li, 2000). Selective law enforcement is often contingent upon

Table 3.1 Summary of the Modes of Hospital Violence

Modes of action	No	Percentage
Non-violent (*wennao*)	82	52.9
Violent (*wunao*)	124	80
Both	51	32.9
No. of participants		
Individual	76	49
Small	31	20
Large	48	31
Results		
Legal Penalty	71	46
Administrative Penalty	37	24
No Punishment	45	29
Others	2	1
Casualties from hospital violence		
Death and Severe Injury	20	13
Minor Injury/No Injury	120	77
NA	15	10
Total	*155*	*100*

the lawbreakers' social status, the disruption level, and the outcomes' severity (Table 3.1).

3.4.2.1 From Concession to Legal Sanction

Based on media reports of 155 medical harassment cases, this study traces the associated penalties and illustrates how selective punishment is implemented by local officials in China. Overall, three levels of punishment are associated with hospital violence—legal penalties (*xingshi chufa*), administrative penalties (*xingzheng chufa*), and no punishment. In the dataset, less than half (46%) of cases received legal penalties, indicating that front-line officials widely adopted concession and selective law enforcement in dealing with hospital violence.

No punishment refers to disruptive protesters receiving concessions and is applied in two circumstances: (1) the people creating the disturbance have low social status or are from vulnerable groups, or (2) the disruptions are small-scale and tolerable. Nearly 30% of disruptive acts—including kneeling, voicing insults, displaying coffins in public spaces, and blocking public roads—did not result in punishment. Despite hospital disruptions being criminalized, front-line local officials often responded passively to disruptive actions.

During my fieldwork, police and other front-line government officials expressed concern about punishing patients or their families, especially those from vulnerable social status. Instead, they showed leniency, attempting to comfort and persuade patients rather than punish them. The sympathy elicited by powerless patients could also explain the government's under-punishment approach; local officials commonly treat the disruptions such patients initiate as disputes rather than crimes; at the street level, front-line police officers are not motivated to intervene in such "social" disputes. One police officer reported addressing dozens of medical disputes monthly, usually sympathizing with the patients:

> In cases of hospital violence organized by individuals that do not lead to severe outcomes, leniency is commonly practiced. We do not want patients to feel that the police only favor the interests of public hospitals. Most of our efforts nowadays emphasize dealing with [incidents as] disputes rather than crimes.[29]

On the one hand, governmental under-punishment could be explained by the less disruptive nature of the patients' acts. Adopting non-violent or less violent behaviors in hospitals is more likely to be met with leniency by local officials. For instance, on 10 October 2016, a mother in a Sichuan hospital waited fifty minutes for her son to receive treatment for a bone fracture. She attempted to communicate with a nurse but felt offended by their indifferent attitude and kicked them. The nurse fought back, and the police and a local juridical worker intervened. After mediation throughout the afternoon and overnight, the two parties (the mother and nurse) agreed that the mother would apologize to the nurse, pay them 2000 RMB in compensation, and not receive further penalties (Case No. 49). Leniency is more often granted when actions are less disruptive to resolve disputes efficiently without agitating patients.

On the other hand, patients are often deemed vulnerable in their power relations with doctors, given the asymmetry of their circumstances. Activists' unfavorable social-economic status arouses public sympathy, and government concessions and tolerance of their disruptive actions are expected. This sympathy towards patients and their relatives legitimates their violent behaviors as a vulnerable group's final resort in seeking justice, depicting threatening or harassing a doctor as an expression of discontent rather than a crime. Chinese cultural understandings of right and wrong deem punishing patients "cruel," and doing so may trigger popular discontent. Therefore, local officials often use persuasion and negotiation with patients and their families to settle medical disputes rather than resort to legal punishments.

Administrative punishment is a symbolic government penalty for disruptive actions, applied in 24% of hospital violence cases. While rules-based, it is tempered by public opinion and organizational pressure.

First, administrative penalties are often applied when lawbreakers are citizens with higher social status. The "legitimation" of hospital disruption is reserved for the weak and less disruptive behaviors. If patients do not belong to this social category, the patient-doctor power asymmetry becomes fundamentally adverse. For instance, when rule breakers are political cadres, the nature of the power asymmetry and public

[29] Interview with the public security officer in the C city, September 2016.

opinion fundamentally change. In Nanjing, Y (case no. 17) was a government official whose 24-year-old daughter was undergoing treatment in a public hospital. A male patient was transferred into her daughter's ward at night, and the bed arrangement in the mixed-gender ward made Y's daughter uncomfortable. She called her mother and asked her parents to negotiate with the nurses to move her to a different ward. The nurse refused because there were no other available beds. Feeling offended, Y struck the nurse on the back and waist with her umbrella. News of the incident spread quickly through the media, and a week later, Y was dismissed from her position due to public pressure. Similarly, a People's Congress representative from Zhangye who beat a doctor was dismissed under public pressure. When the person instigating hospital violence is a political official or powerful figure, it can easily give rise to a "reversal" of public opinion, resulting in support for medical workers and public discontent with political figures who do not abide by the law. Leniency is more often shown when the citizens involved are from vulnerable social groups, while people with higher social statuses or from political cadres more often receive punishment when instigating hospital violence to invite popular pressure and address personal grievances.

Administrative penalties are also applied in cases involving organized protests. As discussed, patients have high mobilizing capacity, and street-level officials must be cautious in dealing with large-scale collective actions. In total, 21 cases involving petitioners on a large scale did not receive any form of punishment, 10 drew administrative penalties, and only 17 large-scale hospital violence cases led to legal penalties. However, nearly all punishments were limited to leaders and key activists. For instance, when relatives surrounded a hospital in a medical dispute in Eastern China, local officials soon arrived and dispersed the group, persuading its members to leave the hospital and detaining the organizer, the only participant to be penalized. In cases where patients are organized by kinship and social ties, it is difficult to punish everyone involved as it could easily induce collective actions. The larger the protest, the less likely everyone will be punished; leaders generally receive symbolic punishment, and the remaining participants are shown leniency.

Administrative penalties are more often applied when hospitals vigorously protect their medical staff's interests. In Shenzhen Hospital (affiliated with Hong Kong University), one mother kicked a nurse because she felt her baby had waited too long for treatment (Case No. 20).[30] The woman received an administrative penalty. She was detained for ten days, even though hospitals often negotiate privately with lawbreakers in similar incidents rather than resort to law. The woman was very annoyed at the penalty she received, saying, "What a big joke that the nurses in the hospital affiliated with Hong Kong University are masters (大爷), incredible!" The strict law enforcement was partially attributed to organizational pressure from the hospital, which cooperated with the local public security office to deter disruptive actions in public institutions. The involved hospital adopted a zero-tolerance

[30] See, for instance, Can Hong Kong Practices be the cure to the medical disputes in Mainland", http://zqb.cyol.com/html/2015-07/22/nw.D110000zgqnb_20150722_2-09.htm, accessed on September 25, 2023.

policy against hospital violence, eschewing private negotiation in favor of strict law enforcement to punish law-breaking behaviors and maintain hospital security and order.

In tackling hospital violence, local officials must balance patients' grievances and the hospitals' interests, accommodating various stakeholders' expectations and demands (Oliver, 1991). Front-line officials must constrain their use of legal sanctions that might motivate angry patients to undertake collective actions while protecting hospitals' authority and healthcare professionals' safety. In some cases, they punish the leaders of disruptive actions to satisfy hospitals' expectations while avoiding punishing all participants to avoid arousing public criticism or agitating the patients.

On the other hand, in cases that arouse wide criticism towards patients and support healthcare professionals, front-line officials tend to take a harsher stance and punish lawbreakers to curry public favor. Conflicting goals motivate them to apply a balanced approach that accommodates the interests of hospitals and doctors, leading to selective punishment. Therefore, a symbolic administrative penalty is applied in cases involving non-violent disruptive acts, large-scale protests, and political cadres who may trigger public opinion.

Third, legal punishment only occurs when unavoidable and is primarily associated with high-violence incidents, such as those resulting in death or significant injury to doctors or nurses. A "red line" is triggered in such incidents, and strict law enforcement is expected. The case pool documents 71 cases of legal punishment for hospital violence incidents; 17 of the 19 cases involving medical workers' death or severe injury resulted in legal punishment.

3.4.2.2 Selective Punishment

Selective punishment has emerged as a common management strategy employed by local officials who punish patients based on the number of protesters, the disruptive tactics involved, and the potential for involving public opinion. The instances of selective punishment described in the previous scenarios share many similarities. Selective punishment is applied in three circumstances: (1) when the people creating disturbances have moral power due to their lower social status or membership in vulnerable groups; (2) when disruptions are small-scale and tolerable; and (3) when disruptions have less severe outcomes. Selective enforcement of the law is common practice in cases of hospital violence. Government intervention is more likely when there is strong public or institutional pressure on doctors and severe violations of the law. Leniency is primarily shown provided the non-compliant behaviors do not severely violate the law (i.e., lead to death or major injury). What matters is not the regulation or law but whether their treatment satisfies public perceptions of morality.

Despite their increased vigilance towards bottom-up resistance, Chinese authorities do not consider repression their only choice; instead, they adopt an array of covert repressive strategies, including channeling and concession, to maintain social stability. Extant scholarship suggests that government responses are largely contingent upon the nature of citizens' claims. For instance, Lee and Hsing (2009) divided citizens' claims when applying resistance into two types: distribution politics and recognition politics. The former involves the pursuit of material interests by various social groups, such as laid-off workers, veterans, and peasants, and is more likely to win concessions from local government. The other concerns the politics of recognition, involving lawyers advocating for women's, migrant workers', and others' rights, and is more likely to prompt direct government repression due to the ideological threat attached. Chen Xi (2020) further supplemented the typology by further differentiating between civic and non-civic behaviors to examine various government responses, finding that civic activism promoting general societal well-being rather than individuals' narrow interests is more likely to draw harsh government intervention.

In dealing with hospital violence, the government's hands are often tied in several ways. On the one hand, patients' claims are non-civic and often based on narrowly defined personal interests; therefore, government concessions are often foreseeable. On the other hand, patients apply disruptive action to force hospitals to take them seriously or gain leverage in bargaining with the government, not to challenge the regime's legitimacy. On the contrary, they form a symbiotic relationship with the government, relying on its legitimacy and benevolence to address their grievances. However, this is not the whole story. A less examined dimension is the claims' morality. The claims informing hospital violence are not just economic or material in nature; they are also emotion-laden narratives designed to arouse others' moral projection, which is more likely to win concession and constrain the use of repression.

In the case of hospital violence, morality is often associated with the vulnerable status of the citizens participating in the rightful resistance. Patients' pitiable status could easily elicit sympathy from the government and public, shielding them from harsh repression. For instance, Yu (2012) found that local police showed a high degree of tolerance and sympathy towards collective actions to advance the compensation claims made by hemophilia patients infected with HIV/AIDS through blood transfusions. Fairly speaking, patients' claims often receive cultural understanding that justifies their disruptive actions in hospitals. In the face of such moral pressure, selective punishment remains a common choice for local officials, who treat incidences of hospital violence as disputes rather than crimes. From their perspective, punishing vulnerable patients does not solve the underlying problem and might backfire, escalating the incident, irritating patients, and causing them to make further trouble. When disruptions are small and initiated by the powerless, government intervention and patient punishment are less likely.

From an interactive perspective, the moral factor shapes the government's selective punishment responses towards disruptive actions. The search for morality is not uncommon in collective actions, often acting as a catalyst (Edelman, 2005). The moral aspects of collective actions are associated with claims and grievances raised by the underprivileged in society, like the peasants' collective action (Feeny, 1983). For instance, Thompson (1971) posed that profiteering in the market dominated citizens' needs, arguing that moral economy refers to psychological processes and stating, "The deep emotions stirred by death, the claims the crowd makes upon authorities ... impart a particular moral charge to the protests." Likewise, Scott (1977) suggested that protesters (especially peasants) act based on their normative view of the world and that norm violation can lead to moral outrage and riots. As Jasper (1997) and Goodwin et al. (2001) studied, collective actions are often born out of "moral shock," which draws disconnected bystanders together and politicizes them. The protesters' morality fuels collective actions and shapes how the government responds.

In cases of hospital violence, patients' and peasants' conceptions of justice are not dissimilar, since lost lives resonate with and affect both. The deaths and injuries of loved ones are not only sources of anger; they also demonstrate patients' decreasing trust in the existing system and belief that it will help them realize their interests, reflect their perceptions of justice, and punish wrongdoers. In hospital violence, patients often couch their claims in the language of morality to arouse others' empathy and moral indignation to protect themselves from repression and sanctions. Per Fesmire (2003), protesters' moral frames arouse "empathetic projection," i.e., putting others in your shoes. Arousing street-level officials' emotional imagination elicits their affection, amplifies patients' bargaining power when negotiating with hospitals or local government, and constrains the government's use of repression and penalty, as local officials and government have a moral responsibility to remedy their grievances.

It is also necessary to note that claims of hospital violence reveal a hybrid type of narrative combining moral, civic, and material claims. One common framing tactic adopted by protesters is ambiguity. Patients' claims are not irrational or spontaneous but involve careful, cost-efficient calculation. For instance, as Hurst (2004) showed, collective actions organized by laid-off workers from state-owned enterprises in Northern China often applied Maoist ideology to advance their pension-related claims. In cases of hospital violence, disputants often use the language of morality to enhance their claims, emphasizing their pursuit of justice (*gong-dao*) rather than their desire for economic compensation, as direct monetary requests would make them appear venal. Despite adopting narratives of rights or justice, patients' claims may still, at their core, be realistic or materialistic. For instance, in the "open letter" case discussed in Chapter One, the patient's family blamed the hospital for its failure to save the lives of their beloved family members. They applied empathy-arousing narratives to elicit moral indignation and simultaneously justify their less obvious monetary compensation requests. Protesters often carefully frame their narrative so that their monetary requests seem to be a by-product of their rights-related claims.

3.4.3 Self-protection Strategies of Hospitals

In the year following the consolidation of the integrated stability maintenance system to address hospital violence through selective law enforcement, doctors still found themselves uneasy about the collaboration and unwilling to trust in it. For instance, a recent empirical study by Huang Xian (2021) finds that the criminalization of hospital violence decreased the public's trust in healthcare professionals and confidence in hospitals' competence and increased their doubts about China's insufficient healthcare system.

Likewise, frequent media reports of hospital violence failed to improve doctors' sense of security and bred their dissatisfaction with the health system. When asked whether they felt safer due to government efforts at making public hospitals guarded, doctors expressed concerns about the weak implementation of the law. Most interviewees indicated that they would rather call on internal security forces, even though patients may see them as the hospital's "black gang." Commenting on his impressions of the public security authority, one interviewee said

> The police often treat them (patients) as a disadvantaged group. We (doctors) have become the scapegoat for an inefficient health system.[31]

Another added,

> They (police) do not undertake sufficient actions to combat hospital violence because they perceive that patients have the right to express their grievances because they have lost loved ones. They fail to protect the safety of the doctors.[32]

As a remedy, hospitals have invested a great deal in security infrastructure to establish connections with public security and have spent much time and effort establishing sound relations with the media to change public opinion. Hospitals have increasingly avoided relying solely on "formal" strategies to address hospital workplace violence, believing their own strategies may allow them to better cope with crises. Some indicated that they did not totally trust the public security authority to protect them. Informal strategies have been increasingly initiated and developed by health professionals, and when hospital violence occurs, health professionals are inclined to seek internal help. These self-protection strategies vary in format but include establishing internal security teams and preparing compensation funds,[33] among others.[34]

According to the government's opinion on strengthening hospitals' safety systems, every 20 hospital beds require one security guard. In reality, most hospitals have done much more. For instance, Zhengzhou City, in Henan Province, established an "armed security team" equipped with helmets, shields, and explosion-proof outerwear to fight and deter hospital violence.[35] Likewise, in another example, a half-dozen people formed an internal security force, the Internal 110,[36] to provide "a sense of security" to hospitals by responding quickly and more efficiently to hospital violence than

---

[31] Interviews with several doctors in C city, January 2017.

[32] Ibid.

[33] For example, doctors could extract a certain percentage of their wages and establish a fund for potential compensation.

[34] Summarized by the author through interviews with several doctors in C city, January 2017, and W city, July 2017.

[35] See, for instance, Zhengzhou organizes "armed security" to fight "medical disturbances". Can it solve the symptoms and root causes? http://news.cntv.cn/special/spj/wuzhuangbaoanzhanyinao/index.shtml, accessed on September 22, 2023.

[36] 110 refers to the emergency contact number in Mainland China.

public security forces did.[37] Hospitals installed new CCTV surveillance systems connected to the public security authority. Based on the author's observations in one public hospital, internal security teams were highly efficient, arriving at disputes within three minutes.

Hospitals and doctors can also collectively settle compensation issues internally. Doctors commonly negotiate privately with patients to avoid career-killing blemishes on their reputations and records. In most cases, the compensation is paid jointly by the department (*yuan* 院), the office (*keshi* 科室), and the individual doctor. The department and office bear the majority of the expense, while the involved doctor's share is deducted from their salary or bonuses. Several doctors admitted that they were unwilling to contact a third-party mediator because they "wanted to keep a clean, professional record"[38] or believed private negotiation through the hospital administrative channel would be more efficient and better serve their interests. Several interviewees reported that they felt local courts were inefficient or unreliable; hence, they would adopt internal strategies rather than seek the cooperation of outside local or state authorities.

In addition to infrastructure renovation and upgrading, medical workers have also applied covert "avoidance" or defensive strategy (He, 2014) in dealing with "high-risk" patients. Similar interviewee accounts reported that they had learned to identify potentially risky patients, even at first glance. For example, some patients carry recording pens to record the doctor's every word without consent. Doctors have become very cautious about treating this type of patient, often discharging them to avoid getting into trouble. The director of one children's hospital's social worker department told the author how to identify potential troublemakers in hospitals:

> For instance, if the patient refuses any treatment advice from medical workers, it often raises a red flag that they do not trust doctors. If the patient asks the medical worker to provide any form of oral commitment, it often suggests that the patient will not accept risk. If the doctor feels the patient is hostile towards doctors, they inform us (social workers) to make a record. We often dispatch our internal social worker to approach the patient and avoid troubles.[39]

During the treatment, the doctors must not only consider their patient's health condition but also their family background, economic burden, and attitudes. For instance, for patients with economic burdens, experienced doctors often manage their expectations proactively by recognizing the possibility of losing both the patient and money due to uncertainty.[40] As one doctor commented, "Every surgery has risks. If I feel that the patient or their family members cannot trust us, I cannot risk performing the surgery."[41] As a preventive strategy to avoid getting into trouble, doctors perform periodic follow-up checks of "high-risk" patients. Some legal experts have suggested that hospitals set up internal blacklists to alert doctors to be cautious when dealing

---

[37] Interviews with several doctors in C city, January 2017.

[38] Ibid.

[39] Interview with the director of social worker department in one tertiary hospital in C city, on August 2022.

[40] Based on author's fieldnote.

[41] Interviews with several doctors in C city, January 2017.

with patients with a "record" of used hospital violence or troublemakers.[42] In other words, doctors are proactively attempting to protect themselves from hospital violence by cherry-picking their patients and performing post-treatment checks on "high-risk" patients.

3.5 Summary

This chapter has categorized and theorized the modes of hospital violence as a form of resistance and traced the inconsistent government strategies used to address disruptive actions in hospitals. Hospital violence is a form of popular resistance that patients apply to protect their rights and seek monetary compensation. This new type of social conflict posits high mobilization power, threatens the social order, and holds the potential to quickly evolve into mass incidents and threaten the trustworthiness, reliability, and legitimacy of public institutions and professional elites in China.

Although the government has launched the Safe Hospital Project and criminalized hospital violence, selective punishment is often applied. The morality embedded in patients' claims has tied the government's hands in dealing with medical disputes. This study contributes to our understanding of various government measures for dealing with rightful resistance in China. It finds that leniency is largely shown to citizens with lower social status and when hospital disruptions are small-scale and tolerable, showing a political and legal tolerance of law-breaking behaviors. It is unfair to say that local officials have not tried to protect doctors' rights and maintain social order in public spaces; however, this chapter has exposed officials' conflicting street-level goals—i.e., simultaneously upholding public morality, social stability, and the law.

This chapter has exposed China's inconsistent street-level law enforcement in cases of hospital violence. By showing leniency in social disputes, officials satisfy the public's demand for "eye-for-an-eye" justice, helping them cope with public pressure, gain popular support, and avoid blame from the masses while affording them flexibility in maintaining social stability. However, selective punishment has also led to the under-enforcement of the law, encouraging the use of non-compliant behaviors. In the long run, selective punishment leads to further disturbances in the social order, a deterioration in patient-doctor relations, and violations of the legal consensus among Chinese citizens.

The underlying reasons for medical disputes and hospital violence remain unaddressed through legal channels. Every incident of hospital violence is associated with sadness, misfortune, and anger. Most acts of extreme violence against medical workers have long histories and are preventable. For instance, patient Lian, who caused one death and two injuries in Wenling, had complained to the hospital for a

[42] See, for instance, Beijing legislates to provide solutions for hospital safety by granting medical staff the "right to avoid risks", https://www.bj148.org/ztk/2021zt/bjzfw2020fzxwhg/xwhg/202101/t20210128_1596947.html, accessed on September 22, 2023.

year before the crime was committed but did not arouse enough attention or assistance. His name and age were incorrect in various patient documents, and Lian felt the hospital had consciously withheld information from him to protect its face.[43] Earlier interventions and medical preventive mechanisms or protocols should be designed to prevent such oversights and serious violations of the law.

Moral indignation and the power asymmetry between patients and hospitals motivated patients to adopt hospital violence as a form of resistance to protect their rights. The lack of channels for patients to address their disputes and the system's ineffective legal responses have given rise to mediation channels and the routinization and institutionalization of social dispute resolution in China, as will be discussed in the next two chapters.

References

Blom, A., & Jaoul, N. (2008) Introduction. The moral and affectual dimension of collective action in South Asia. *South Asia Multidisciplinary Academic Journal*, (2) URL: http://journals.openedition.org/samaj/1912. https://doi.org/10.4000/samaj.1912

Bo, S., Chen, J., Song, Y., & Zhou, S. (2020) Media attention and choice of major: Evidence from anti-doctor violence in China. *Journal of Economic Behavior & Organization*, *170*: 1–19.

Chen, F. (2003) Between the state and labour: The conflict of Chinese trade unions' double identity in market reform. *The China Quarterly*, 176: 1006–1028.

Chen, X. (2020) Civic and noncivic activism under autocracy: shifting political space for popular collective action. *Mobilization: An International Quarterly*, *25*(SI): 623–640.

Chen, C. J., & Cai, Y. (2021) Upward targeting and social protests in China. Journal of Contemporary China, 30(130): 511–525.

Chhabra, N., & Houser, S. M. (2009) The diagnosis and management of empty nose syndrome. *Otolaryngologic Clinics of North America*, *42*(2): 311–330.

Chiu Yuchan. (2007) "Yibing xingxiang de meiti jiangou —yiliaojiufen taiguankangyi xinwen fenxi" ("The media depiction of images of doctors and patients-An analysis of news coverage of coffin-lifting resulting from medical dispute ")*(Mass Communication Research),(93)*: 41–81.

Davenport, C. (1995) Multi-dimensional threat perception and state repression: An inquiry into why states apply negative sanctions. *American Journal of Political Science*: 683–713.

Du Zhichun (2015) "Zhongguo shehui gong anquan yanjiu baogao" (Report on Chinese social public security research), (Central Compilation & Translation Press).

Duncan, L. E. (1999) Motivation for collective action: Group consciousness as mediator of personality, life experiences, and women's rights activism. *Political Psychology*, *20*(3), 611–635.

Edelman, M. (2005) Bringing the moral economy back in… to the study of 21st-century transnational peasant movements. *American anthropologist*, *107*(3): 331-345.

Fang, P. (2015) China Healthcare Development Report 2014: Bejing: Renmin Press.

Feeny, D. (1983) The moral or the rational peasant? Competing hypotheses of collective action. *The Journal of Asian Studies*, *42*(4): 769-789.

Feng, Y., & Zeng, Y. (2022) Stability justice: Petitioners versus non-petitioners in China's criminal adjudication. *Law & Society Review*, *56*(4): 555–579.

[43] See, for instance, A bloody case involving doctors and patients with no winners: Reflections on the doctor-killing case in Wenling, Zhejiang, http://politics.people.com.cn/n/2014/0127/c70731-24245553.html, accessed on September 22, 2023.

Fesmire, S. (2003) *John Dewey and moral imagination: Pragmatism in ethics*. Indiana University Press.

Goffman, E. (2017) *Interaction ritual: Essays in face-to-face behavior*. Routledge.

Goodwin, J., Jasper, J. M., & Polletta, F. (Eds.) (2001) *Passionate politics: Emotions and social movements*. University of Chicago Press.

Gould, R. V. (1991) Multiple networks and mobilization in the Paris Commune, 1871. *American Sociological Review*,:716–729.

Habermas, J. (1990) *Moral consciousness and communicative action*. MIT press.

Hanser, A. (2016) Street politics: Street vendors and urban governance in China. *The China Quarterly*, *226*: 363-382.

He, A. J. (2014) The doctor–patient relationship, defensive medicine and overprescription in Chinese public hospitals: Evidence from a cross-sectional survey in Shenzhen city. *Social science & medicine, 123*: 64–71.

Huang, X. (2021) Peace in the Shadow of Unrest: yinao and the State Response in China. *The China Quarterly*, *247*: 724–748.

Hurst, W. (2004) Understanding contentious collective action by Chinese laid-off workers: the importance of regional political economy. *Studies in Comparative International Development*, *39*: 94–120.

Jasper, J. M. (1997) *The art of moral protest*. University of Chicago Press.

Jasper, J. M., & Poulsen, J. D. (1995) Recruiting strangers and friends: Moral shocks and social networks in animal rights and anti-nuclear protests. *Social problems*, *42*(4): 493-512.

Lee, C. K., & Hsing, Y. T. (2009) Social activism in China: Agency and possibility. In *Reclaiming Chinese Society* (pp. 13–26) Routledge.

Li Peilei, & Deng Yong. (2015) "Yiliao Jiufen 'xian'e siliao' tiaokuan pingjia ji gaijin jianyi" ("Policy Evaluation and Recommendation on the "pricing limit for the private negotation" in medical dispute resolution") *(Chinese Health Policy Research)*, *8*(9), 45–52.

Liebman, B. L. (2013) Malpractice mobs: medical dispute resolution in China. *Columbia Law Review*: 181–264.

Liu, J., Zhou, H., Liu, L., & Wang, C. (2020) The weakness of the strong: examining the squeaky-wheel effect of hospital violence in China. *Social Science & Medicine*, *245*, 112717.

Luo, J., Liu, H., Liu, Y., Jiang, F., & Tang, Y. L. (2021) The association between medical liability insurance coverage medical disturbances in tertiary psychiatric hospitals in china: a national survey. Risk Management and Healthcare Policy:3767–3774.

Luttrell, J. C. (2019) *White people and Black Lives Matter: Ignorance, empathy, and justice*. Springer.

McCarthy, J. D., & Zald, M. N. (1977) Resource mobilization and social movements: A partial theory. *American journal of sociology*, *82*(6): 1212–1241.

McDonald, A. F. (2019) Framing# MeToo: Assessing the power and unintended consequences of a social media movement to address sexual assault. *Handbook of sexual assault and sexual assault prevention*: 79–107.

Milcent, C. (2016) Evolution of the Health System. Inefficiency, Violence, and Digital Healthcare. *China perspectives*, *2016*(2016/4): 39–50.

O'brien, K. J., & Li, L. (2000) Accommodating "democracy" in a one-party state: Introducing village elections in China. *The China Quarterly*, *162*: 465–489.

Oliver, C. (1991) Strategic responses to institutional processes. *Academy of management review*, *16*(1): 145–179.

Parkinson, S. E. (2013) Organizing rebellion: Rethinking high-risk mobilization and social networks in war. *American Political Science Review*, *107*(3), 418–432.

Scott, J. C. (1977) *The moral economy of the peasant: Rebellion and subsistence in Southeast Asia* (Vol. 315) Yale University Press.

Scott, J. C. (1985) *Weapons of the weak: Everyday forms of peasant resistance*. Yale University Press.

Snow, D. A., Zurcher Jr, L. A., & Ekland-Olson, S. (1980) Social networks and social movements: A microstructural approach to differential recruitment. *American sociological review*: 787–801.
Snyder-Reinke, J. (2016) Afterlives of the Dead: Uncovering Graves and Mishandling Corpses in Nineteenth-Century China. *Frontiers of History in China, 11*(1): 1–20.
Thompson, E. P. (1971) The moral economy of the English crowd in the eighteenth century. *Past & present*, (50): 76–136.
Tucker, J. D., Cheng, Y., Wong, B., Gong, N., Nie, J. B., Zhu, W., & Kleinman, A. (2015) Patient–physician mistrust and violence against physicians in Guangdong Province, China: a qualitative study. *BMJ open*, *5*(10), e008221.
Van Stekelenburg, J. (2013) Moral incentives. In *The Wiley-Blackwell Encyclopedia of Social and Political Movements* (pp. 770–771) Wiley-Blackwell.
Van Stekelenburg, J., Klandermans, B., & Van Dijk, W. W. (2009) Context matters: Explaining how and why mobilizing context influences motivational dynamics. *Journal of Social Issues*, *65*(4), 815–838.
Wahlström, M., Peterson, A., & Wennerhag, M. (2018) "Conscience Adherents" Revisited: Non-Lgbt Pride Parade Participants. *Mobilization: An International Quarterly*, 23(1), 83–100.
Wiles, D. (2001) *Freedom summer*. Simon and Schuster.
Yu Zhiyuan. (2012) "jitixing kangzheng xingdong jieguo de yingxiang yinsu _yixiang jiyu sange jitixing kangzhengxingdong de bijiaoyanjiu" ("The Factors Shaping the Outcomes of Collective Actions: A comparative study on three collective action cases") *(Sociological Studies)*, (3): 90–112.

Chapter 4
The Art of Persuasion: Everyday Mediation Practice

因事之理，则不劳而成。
Following the patterns (li) of the heavens, then things could be achieved without effort.
—韩非子《外储说右下》*Han Fei Zi [A collection of Saying VI].*

This chapter examines the rise of the People's Mediation in dealing with the rising medical disputes as well as absorbing social grievances. Drawing on ethno-graphic fieldwork in people's mediation, I explained why and how the mediators have addressed social grievances in an efficient manner and achieve political and social goals simultaneously. I find that the mediation process was full of power interactions. Specifically, I summarize a series of mediators' daily practices and theorize it as politicization, affective and bargaining strategies, which discourage and deter the (potential) collective actions, satisfy the disputants' psychological demands and provide monetary compensation to settle the case respectively. By doing so, it jointly led to the high mediation success rate. This chapter enhances our understanding of the adaptive role of the People's Mediation channel from an institutional perspective and contributes to crystalizing the dynamical strategies in the mediation process.

The earlier version of this Chapter, Jie Wu, "Specialty Mediation Committees for Medical Disputes in China", *China: An International Journal* 19, no. 4 (November 2021): 166–187. 10.1353/chn.2021.0046 was published by "China: An International Journal", East Asian Institute, National University of Singapore. The author thanks the East Asian Institute for allow me to reusing part of the article.

See, for instance, Chinese Text Project of the Hundred Schools of Thought in Pre-Qin and Han, https://ctext.org/hanfeizi/wai-chu-shuo-you-xia/ens, accessed on September 30, 2023.

J. Wu, *Politicized Medical Dispute Resolution in China*, Understanding China,
https://doi.org/10.1007/978-981-97-6961-2_4

4.1 Introduction

As illustrated in the previous Chapter, the selective implementation of law failed to address the disputes, nor restore the social order in health institutions. Hence, since the 2010s, the Chinese government has revitalized the traditional People's Mediation Channels to absorb patients' grievances, address medical disputes, as well as maintain social stability, which has achieved great success. According to the Ministry of Justice, from 2010 to 2017, there were 3,565 people's mediation committees established as the venue for medical dispute resolution which staffed with over 20, 000 mediators. As such, 60 per cent of the medical disputes have been channelled from the courtroom, the street, and the hospital into the mediation channel, and reached an 85 per cent success rate.[1]

Such high success rate prompted us to wonder: What are the routinized approaches for the mediators in dealing with medical disputes? How do mediators persuade the disputants? What tactics do they apply to convince the grieved disputant to reconcile with the hospitals? In this Chapter, I examine the everyday practice of mediation and summarize an array of the strategies that mediation applied to persuade two involved parties—disputants as well as the hospital representatives. During this process, mediators are the key intermediary between the hospital and patients to facilitate the reconciliation process, which changed the power asymmetry between the doctors and patients.

Drawing on intensive ethnographic fieldwork in the mediation committees, I find that the mediators are sophisticated in employing politicization, affective, as well as bargaining strategies to satisfy stability maintenance goals but also meet disputants' psychological needs and promote consistent decisions. The dispute resolution through the mediation channel could not only gather the local information to prevent the occurrence of collective actions but also neutralize the disputant's claim to dissolve their heightened emotion.

First, in medical dispute resolution, the foremost issue is to maintain social stability. With the party-state's promotion of mediation channels in social dispute resolution, the novel people's mediation institutions have gradually gained a high degree of proficiency and formalism. While in addition to the routinized procedure for the mediators to intervene in the medical dispute resolution process, mediators remain flexible to give priority to difficult cases that have a higher possibility of attracting unwanted public attention or involving disruptive actions. The mediators often pursue a graduated control strategy by allocating more time for difficult cases. For instance, cases that would have the potential to lead or have already led to escalating into collective actions would be given the most priority. Meanwhile, cases that involve children or disadvantaged social groups would also warrant more attention, since these cases may attract unwanted media attention and arouse public empathy or moral indignation. In addition, the working calendar of the mediation committees

---

[1] See, for instance, More than 60% of medical disputes in China are resolved through people's mediation, with a success rate of 85%, http://www.xinhuanet.com/politics/2019-02/15/c_1124116833.htm, accessed on September 30, 2023.

also synthesized with and reflected the government's preference. For instance, during crucial timing such as National Holidays, People's Congress meetings, and Party's Congress conferences, the mediation committee would devote more attention and report to the local health bureau and juridical office if there involved tough cases. In dealing with special cases, mediators proactively aligned with the local government to address the social stability concerns by resorting to discretional power and flexible governance.

Compared to other dispute resolution channels such as courtrooms, mediation required more devotion of time and effort from the mediators. In practice, one or two mediator(s) are assigned and shoulder responsibility for the case from end to end. This institutional design allows mediators to allocate more time to communicate with the disputants and develop emotional ties with the disputants, aiming to smooth the resolution process. For medical dispute cases, disputants are sometimes deeply influenced by intense emotions. Mediators, different from judges, are expected not only to address disputes in a timely manner but also to untie the knot in one's heart (打开心结), which is believed could address the dispute from its origin and win the trust of the disputant. Mediators spend great efforts in providing psychological consulting, affective care, and persuasion with the disputants to establish authority and win the disputants' trust. It also reflected a new trend in dispute resolution—the increasing use of affective governance which refers to the party-state's mobilizing and regulating citizens' emotions to solicit disputants' consent. Mediators often perform as emotion workers and resort to non-coercive persuasion and communication skills to interact with the disputants, as well as to negotiate with the hospital. Hence, from the government's perspective, dispute cases that went through the mediation channel were better off and less likely to threaten social stability due to the contribution of the mediation, yet few examined the detailed persuasion strategies of the mediators.

The overall study builds on two years of fieldwork in the C city, while observing medical disputes resolution. I conducted 72 in-depth interviews with patients, medical workers, and mediators and reviewed 762 mediated medical disputes cases. Among the dispute cases, the percentage of medical disputes solved through mediation channels ranged from 83 to 93%; only 77 of the 762 cases did not achieve agreement between the hospital and the patient, and 17 cases were transferred to the litigation channel (Fig. 4.1). Nearly 90% of the disputes occurred in public hospitals, and the average amount of compensation for each mediated case was 39,292 RMB in 2017 (equal to 5990 US dollars), sharply dropping from the original mean claim of 170,438 RMB. I found that medical disputes were solved in a highly "efficient" manner: the average mediation duration was approximately thirty days, and patients also agreed to accept a reduced amount of compensation after mediation. Moreover, all cases that went through mediation did not further lead to collective actions. This chapter theorizes the everyday practice in the mediation by unveiling the secret weapon of the mediators.

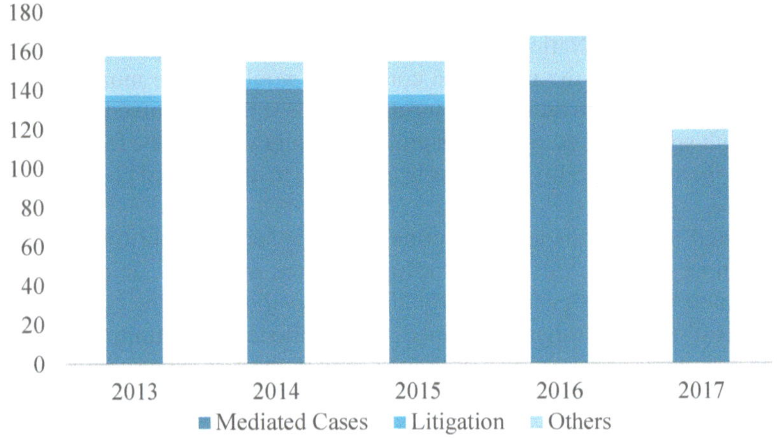

Fig. 4.1 Trend of medical dispute resolution from 2013 to 2017 in the fieldwork city. *Source* Based on author's fieldwork

4.1.1 Standard Operation in Dispute Mediation

What is the institutional design for the people's mediation channel in dealing with medical dispute cases? Fig. 4.2 plots the standardized dispute resolution process. The mediation committee plays a brokerage role in linking patients and hospitals under the liaison of the mediators to communicate and negotiate.

Today, in every district in C city, there is at least one medical dispute mediation committee providing professional service to the needy. The accessibility and economy of the mediation channel are attractive to the disputants, which successfully channels the patients from the courtroom or the street back to the mediation room. At the starting point, the mediators accept cases from two channels. On the

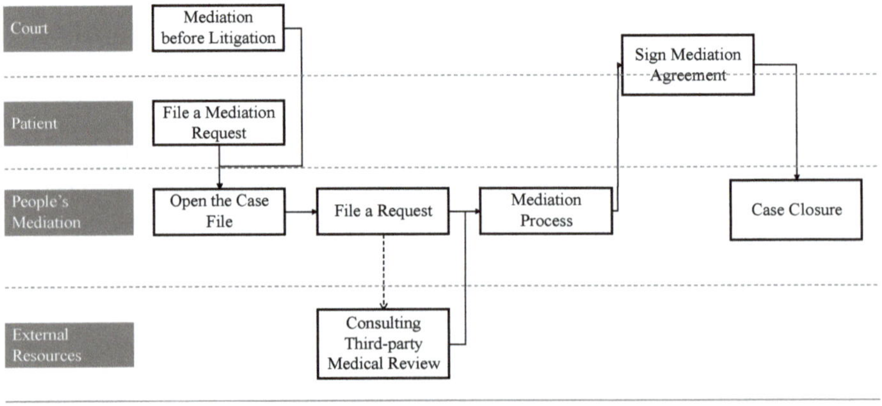

Fig. 4.2 Workflow of the medical mediation committee. *Source* Based on author's fieldwork

one hand, patients could visit the People's mediation committee in person for a case consultation. Many patients find the committee the most convenient and cost-saving channel as the mediation is free of charge. For instance, during the fieldwork, Auntie Zhang visited the people's mediation committee at least three times before she made up her mind to open the case file in the mediation committee I visited. During the interview, she said,

> My husband's orthopedic surgery is unsuccessful and now he finds it hard to walk. You know, the lawyer (I consulted) told me the hospital involved needed to compensate at least one million yuan for my case, but the mediators here told me that the lawyer was not telling me the truth, merely to scam me. The mediator told me that if I was not satisfied with the result, I could still file the lawsuit against the hospital anyway. As the mediation process here is free, what can I lose? So, after three visits, I stayed with the mediation channel to give it a try.[2]

On the other hand, the mediators also accept transferred cases from the government, courtrooms, hospitals, etc. For instance, the hospital's internal office (yuanban 院办) would inform the district-level people's mediation committee when they find it hard to reach a reconciliation with the patient or has a high possibility of encountering hospital violence. Police would also transfer the disputants that apply disruptive actions in health institutions to the mediation channel to seek reconciliation. In those scenarios, the difficulty of these transferred cases is often foreseeable.

In processing the case, the institutional design divides the case to two categories, with various procedures, as differentiating strategy. Dispute with a large compensation request (over 100,000 yuan) has to go through medical technical examination performed by a few selected well-known doctors chosen from the expert pools. The name list of the expert pools is composed of the most distinguished experts in various fields within the district. To avoid the manipulated process, the committee would shield interest conflict by avoiding choosing experts from the same health institution to promote patient trust. In fact, the committee often consult the most well-established and seniority expert in the field as they enjoyed a high social status based on their credentials. The expert review team would reach a conclusion regarding the responsibility attribution in the medical dispute.

Next, the mediators would invite hospital representative and their lawyers, as well as patients to attend the closed-door meetings at the venue of mediation committees. To avoid leaving the impression on the patients that the mediation committee favours their interests with the public institutions, the mediators often sit alongside the patients to show their support. It usually takes at least two or three times before reaching a conclusion. During this, the mediator would keep close contact with the patients and hospital representatives to exchange information and allow patients' express their demands and expectations via personal contacts. The whole mediation process would usually cost 30 days (within a month). In fact, the duration of mediation is often applied as a crucial indicator to measure mediators' performance as it projected the efficacy of the mediation channel compared to the lawsuits. For instance, during the interview, one city-level juridical authority proudly said,

---

[2] Interview with Auntie Zhang in the mediation committee, August 2017.

> We have designated one to two officers for each case. The average processing cycle for each case has shortened from 60 to 30 days. The latest data showed that we solved the majority (70 percent) of the medical disputes within 30 days; to be more detailed, the average processing cycle decreased to 25–27 days in 2016.[3]

The institutional design of the mediation process gave the mediators great motivation to address the dispute case in an efficient manner. It is not surprising that the medical dispute cases would take a long time, due to the complexity of the medical and legal issues and the complex burden-of-proof process. For instance, compared to other types of disputes (e.g., labor disputes), medical disputes receive more media attention and controversy. The average processing time for a medical dispute (from injury to filing a claim) is 1.6 years (with error) and 2.2 years (no error) in the U.S. (Studdert et al., 2006, p. 2030). However, in China, the process lasts only a month (30 days) on average from opening the case to reaching the final agreement in the mediation channel. Such high efficiency has no doubt that motivated the government to prefer mediation channels over legal ones in addressing social disputes. Meanwhile, the high success rate also has promoted us to ask, how do the mediators seek agreement among patients and doctors so efficiently? What's their secret in persuading the disputants who are often with heightened emotions? Next, before depicting the detailed strategies of mediators for both regular and tough cases, I first examined how mediation channels break the power asymmetry through the intermediary role of political- and social-embedded mediators.

4.2 Mediation Channel: Breaking the Power Asymmetry

People's Mediation Committees refer to the semi-government, mass-organized institutions that helped to address social disputes, ranging from interpersonal neighbor conflict to labor and medical disputes that involve expertise and professional knowledge through persuasion and negotiation. Recent scholarship has paid increasing attention to the mediation committees—how they absorb popular grievances, address disputes, and promote social stability. Wall Jr. James and Michael Blum (1991) called China "the most heavily mediated nation on earth". Mediation institutions used to be an innovative way that the Party applied since the Revolutionary era in the Border region, which gradually faded away since the reform and open-up. In face of the social changes, mediation has demonstrated a high level of adaptivity by transforming the old Maoist weapon into the new era. Mediation institutions have experienced profound institutional change by imbuing and packing up new functions to address social disputes. Fairly speaking, today, people's mediation committees not only prioritize conflict resolution to satisfy social control goals but also create specialized mediation committees to promote professionalism in dispute resolution.

[3] Author's interview with an officer from the judicial authority, August 2016.

Why is the mediation channel preferred? Extant studies mainly explained the revival of the People's Mediation institutions in the 2000s from the top-down government's perspective. The study of Zhuang Wenjia and Chen Feng (2015) explained the rationale for the revitalization of mediation from various perspectives by taking the example of labor dispute mediation. Economically, the mediation channel could flexibly uphold the labor standards to limit the amount of compensation and protect the local economy. Politically, mediation works as an alternative means of legal channel in dispute resolution that contributes to social stability maintenance. It also satisfies the managerial rationale by absorbing the disputes that could not be channeled or addressed in the formal institutions. The bureaucratic rationale is also worth noting. For the juridical officials, the mediation channel could contribute to their better performance by avoiding appeals and increasing their success rate of mediation. Similarly, Zhang Jing and Cai Yongshun's study (2019) showed the advent of mediation institutions also helped the local government to avoid blame by shifting the dispute resolution role to the mediators.

Institutionally speaking, faced with the growing complexity of society and the rising occurrence of social disputes, people's mediation has gradually grown in professionalism and sophistication to prioritize not only government interests but also respond to citizens' grievances. The high penetration of the people's mediation committees at the grassroots increased the "visibility" of the government's role in regulating social relations. Like the prior traditional community- or village-based mediation committees, the geographical proximity, accessibility, and high penetration of the mediation institutions allowed the local government to offer instant help to the citizens. It also confined and downsized the dispute to the locality, avoiding the skip-level petitioning activity or "linking up" activities. Meanwhile, in addition to their political embeddedness of mediators, today, these people's mediations have gained high proficiency and specialty by appointing professional mediators to deal with specific types of disputes. It jointly refashioned the people's mediation that was initiated in the traditional era to accommodate the new demands of the social governance.

Though many insights have been gained from the prior literature, few examine the social meaning of mediation from the power perspective, let alone the strategies that mediators undertake in their daily practices. As discussed in the previous Chapters, the power asymmetry between the disputants and public institutions has become the stumbling block that hinders trust in patient-doctor relations. I find that the key to the mediation institutions was to rewrite the power relations in the dispute resolution process. Through the intermediary role of the mediators, it not only provided a safe space between hospitals and patients which divided them physically to prevent the occurrence of disturbances, but also changed their embedded power asymmetry.

The intuitive concept of power, based on Dahl (1957, p. 202–203), is defined as A having power over B to do something that he would not otherwise have done. However, the exercise of power may not directly translate to direct behavior change; it is sometimes linked to compliance through the ability to use sanctions, coercion or authority (Lukes, 1974). Sociologists have further conceptualized power from a social exchange perspective: it is the ability to influence and change one's behavior or make another compliant during the process of social exchange (Baldwin, 1978; Blau, 2017). The exercise of power exists in daily practice and is applied to describe the dynamic social relations among various (at least two) social actors. This study reports how the element of power is exercised in the process of medical malpractice mediation. Specifically, it contextualizes and describes how government-led mediation exercises power over patients and doctors to influence them to accept the dispute mediation results and discourage them from further collective action or bargaining.

The dispute resolution process is not immune to power. Power is a relative concept constrained by time, counterpart, and culture. From the Chinese political and social perspective, a combination of authority and guanxi (social connections) are key factors in assessing power in China (Bian, 1994; Hwang, 1987; Pye & Pye, 2009). Authority is defined by the social hierarchy or position/status in society (Martin, 2002), which is closely associated with power. In Chinese culture, the measurement of authority is based on relations with the government. According to Pye & Pye (2009), any claims to authority that fall outside the structure of government are seen as illegitimate. The formal bureaucratic hierarchy within the political system and government relationships are crucial for evaluating the authority of social actors in the Chinese context. Hence, a relatively higher ranking in a hierarchical society secures more authority. Failure to generate authority over a counterpart may result in an inferior or subordinate position in the power structure. In the medical dispute process, patients often define their position as vulnerable: doctors are protected by the formal institutions, and themselves on the fringe. The introduction of the mediation channels worked as leverage allowing for a balancing of power relations between the hospital and patients.

Doctors, or hospital representatives involved in medical disputes often enjoyed high social professional authority in Chinese societies, especially those in tertiary hospitals. On the one hand, under the "halo effect", knowledgeable persons from prestigious institutions are more effective and persuasive than others and rendering it more trustworthy due to their expertise (Carlson, 2019; Wilson and Sherrel, 1993). Given their expertise, these healthcare professionals as intellectuals could bear high credibility and normative power. On the other hand, doctors have natural connections with the government. Public hospitals are still the mainstream health service providers in China. The most prestigious hospitals in China are the public hospitals in metropolitan cities that share natural political or bureaucratic bonds with the government and are partially financed by the government. Doctors enjoyed a favorable social status given their political connections and professional knowledge.

According to Michelson's study (2007), socially disadvantaged families are more likely to resort to mediation due to their limited access to the legal system, while in comparison, educated urban dwellers may be more likely to turn to lawyers for help. In medical disputes, though the disputants are much more diverse and resourceful compared to those in labor disputes with various goals, they still lack institutional resources to address their grievances. According to the mediators, patients are usually less advantaged in terms of social resources, professional knowledge, and connections. Given the fact that disputants usually lacked professional discourse authority and social connections, holding higher authority in the social hierarchy often put hospitals in a favorable position in seeking compliance from a counterpart with less authority.

The social interactions between doctors and patients are full of the symbol of power exchange in order to seek others' compliance. As such, the social power inequality as well as asymmetry was reproduced in the process. The case of Mr. C would be representative in illustrating the power asymmetric among the doctors and disputants. Mr. C is a migrant worker from a neighboring province with a humble background. He lost his only child in a prestigious children's hospital and was overwhelmed with the feeling of being treated indifferently.

> I was a peasant farmer in Subei (North of Jiangsu Province) with my wife for a living. I have no doubt in their (the hospital's) medical excellence; my son had been treated many times here...The hospital must apologize to me publicly, and the doctors and nurses should be punished. I am not here for money. They should reimburse us all the money that we spent on raising my son.[4]

In his narratives, he emphasized his vulnerable and powerless status in the medical disputes as he was confronting a giant public organization with high authority. Through his emotion-laden narratives, he hoped the hospitals to treat him seriously, as he is powerless and with limited social connections in the mega city. The social inequality between the patient and doctors are exercised and reproduced in dispute resolution process.

However, the introduction of the mediators has helped him change his status, as well as rewritten or reverse the power asymmetry between the patients and doctors. Who are the mediators? According to the regulation on Strengthening the Building of Industry-based and Profession-based People's Mediation Committees in 2011,[5] mediators must have a relevant professional background and expert knowledge of law or have prior experience providing legal services or social work, etc. For instance, medical dispute mediators in the fieldwork city are experts in dispute resolution and acquire professional knowledge related to law, medicine, governance, social work, etc.

Mediators are deeply embedded in the social and political system, rendering high social authority, which made them favored in the mediation process. Embeddedness refers to the behaviors and institutions constrained by ongoing social relations (Granovetter, 2018). Mediators not only manifested official relations with the government authorities but also developed sound social networks with the community. In the fieldwork, 75 per cent of the mediators in medical disputes were employed directly by government organizations, including public hospitals, police bureaus and legal bureaus. For instance, they are often retired police officers and court clerks, who have grasped a certain degree amount of legal knowledge and are deeply embedded in the political system. The mediators are or used to be public personnel and have work experience in public institutions and government organisations; these bureaucratic

[4] Interview with patient C in August 2017.

[5] See, for instance, Opinions of the Ministry of Justice on strengthening the construction of industry-specific and professional people's mediation committees, http://www.12348.gov.cn/pub/12348/ztj/flfg/201803/t20180322_496.html, accessed on September 30, 2023.

ties help the institutions maintain government connections (Huang, 2006). Meanwhile, they have developed sound social networks and trust in the locality. Some mediators were recruited from among full-time professional social workers, who are relatively younger or in their middle age. According to an official from the city's judicial bureau, the mediators need to have a sound understanding of the law; they are also proficient at using sophisticated mediating techniques to persuade the disputants, and they, because of their good moral character, in turn earn the disputants' respect and trust.[6] In other words, mediators in the region are expected to be (i) familiar with tackling and intervening in disruptive actions and troublemaking tactics; (ii) adept at providing basic legal advice and psychological comfort; and (iii) well connected to the health or government system.

The political- and social-embeddedness of the mediators not only facilitated the dispute resolution process, but also largely shaped their strategies. On the one hand, given their political ties, they enjoyed more resources and authority to persuade the disputants as well as the hospitals, under the name of the public. Their political embeddedness also allows them to understand the government's goal and interests in dispute resolution, which set the cornerstone for the mediation process and results. The local government could instrumentally rely on mediators to reflect the government's goal in social stability maintenance and discourage all types of collective actions effectively since mediators are "enmeshed" in the bureaucratic system. On the other hand, the mediators also enjoyed social authority due to their expertise, seniority, and knowledge. The key to the mediation efficacy relies on the capability and resources of the mediators to represent, interact and persuade the disputants. Since the mediation institutions are locality-based, mediators also keep strong ties with the community and are resourceful. It also allows them to persuade and negotiate with the disputants by utilizing their social embeddedness. The dual social- and political-embeddedness of the mediators transformed the mediators into a firm stabilizer in the society, bridging two parties in disputes.

With the help of the mediators, it changed the imbalanced power structure between him and the hospitals by borrowing and bringing external social power and political authority into the interactions between the doctor and patient. Since the mediators are deeply connected with the political system, their presence in the medical dispute resolution would make the powerless disputant break the asymmetric balance and add weight to favoring the rights of disputants. Meanwhile, since the disputants (patients) are vulnerable and pitiable, the mediators often shoulder the affective obligation to provide necessary care and assistance to those types of disputants in the social exchange and interaction process. More importantly, the mediators are also deeply embedded with the government system, which could function as the "extended arm" of the government while avoiding the latter's direct involvement. Since the medical dispute committee is sponsored by the government, external political and social power has been introduced and shaped the way the dispute resolution is carried out, and its outcomes as well. It aimed to change the power asymmetry and promote the fair game between the doctors and patients, under the intermediary role of the

[6] Author's interview with an officer from the judicial authority in August 2017.

mediators. Next, through intensive cases, I summarized the secret to the mediator's success.

4.3 The Art of Mediation

4.3.1 Dynamic Goals and Toolkit of Mediators

In the mediation process, the goals of the grieved patients are complex. Some patients want to proactively protect their rights by suing the doctors, finding the truth of the medical disputes, while others may focus on requesting monetary compensation, or simply vent their dissatisfaction with the hospitals and doctors, etc. Still others may want to punish the doctors involved by adopting disruptive actions (e.g., see Liebman, 2013). Mediators, therefore, have developed three main goals with corresponding varied strategies: (1) to deter disputants and prevent the occurrence of collective actions to maintain the social stability (politicization strategy); (2) to provide social assistance to disputants to absorb social grievances and win the trust of the disputants (affective strategy); and (3) to address medical disputes through channeling them from right protection to compensation bargaining in order to neutralize the nature of medical dispute (economic bargaining). The mediators would either apply the tactic by sequential or use a combination of various tactics collectively. This section discusses each strategy in detail and depicts the toolkits of mediators.

4.3.2 Politicization

The first and utmost goal of the mediators is to maintain social stability and discourage and forbid any chances and occurrences of collective actions, let alone social unrest. Although the medical disputes do not challenge the ruling regime and endanger the core power structure of the government, they instead wield a high degree of moral influence over disputants' deep grievances. Failing to be responsive to the disputants' demands, would easily arouse moral indignation from the public, channeling the target of citizens' anger from involved public institutions to the government authorities. Since the disputants are often emersed with huge grievances, anger, and hate, the connection to resistance and collective actions is rather close (Jasper, 2004, 2011). As discussed, the mediators are selectively recruited from the government authorities (especially policing bureaus), naturally prioritizing government goals in stability maintenance. Hence, mediators often apply the politicization strategy to deter disputants in cases that could possibly lead to collective action.

The politicization strategy involves pre-emptive tactic and coercive approaches (such as sanctions and punishments) to delegitimize and discourage collective actions. Through politicization approach, the mediators could exert political pressures to deter the disputants from engaging in (potential) collective actions and group petitioning, particularly during the politically sensitive time period. From the mediators' perspective, their work began before the collective action could have ever taken place. The following is the case that mediators intervened jointly with the help of multiple government authorities to prevent the occurrence of collective action during the sensitive time period, which also illustrated their politicization tactic and goals.

In September 2017, a group of patients with ankylosing spondylitis (an incurable chronic arthritic disease) were lured by hospital TV commercials to receive unnecessary, yet expensive treatment (approximately RMB15,000 [US$2,322] per course) to alleviate their neck and spine pain by one private hospital located in the city. The doctors in the private hospitals exaggerated the effect of the medical treatment and promised the disease could be curable by receiving high-tech treatment. This "misleading advertisement" of the treatment also diffused across many provinces through television, which attracted the patients across various provinces. However, patients later found that they had been deceived since the treatment alleviated the pain for only a month and did not cure their disease as promised. Feeling being misled and falsified; the patients attempt to organize a group petition to the hospital representatives to get their money back. The patients were located throughout the country, ranging from Liaoning in the northeast China to Xinjiang which located in the western areas, and many of them were disabled, with limited mobility. The geographically dispersed patients made the collective actions difficult to take place and shielded the private hospitals from the organized pressure of the patients. Hence, the private hospital refused to provide any form of compensation and deny the claims of the patients.

At that moment, Mr. A, a disabled person, took the lead,[7] who has once accumulated rich experience in utilizing petitioning channel to protect his right vigorously. Firstly, he formed an online WeChat group (online forum) to overcome the geographical barriers of communication and online mobilization. The online forum became a shared platform for the patients to express their grievances and provided the organizational base for potential collective action. Meanwhile, to boost the patients' bargaining position by mobilizing more patients, he planned to convene people to surround the private hospital jointly the following Monday, 23 October 2017. He talked the patients into organizing as many people as possible as that would be the only way to force the hospitals to compensate them. In addition, to overcome the collective action dilemma of the frequent exit and fragmentation of the participants, the leader of the patient group took advance payment for public transport tickets from patients and then distributed the tickets on the day to ensure their attendance.[8] By doing so, he sought to ensure the patients' attendance and avoid unwanted patients' exit, in order to make a strong presence in front of the target private hospital.

Using this organizational tactic, the patient participants mobilized and agreed to show up. However, the proposed date of the collective action targeting the private

[7] Author's interviews and participatory observation with Mr X, from October to November 2017.

[8] Author's interview with a patient alliance organizer Z, October 2017.

hospital has been coincided with the week of the 19th National Congress of the Communist Party of China (CPC), which they were not quite aware of. During such critical and sensitive political moments, the Chinese authorities are very cautious about grassroots activism, and have applied advanced technologies in censoring and identifying potential risks, especially those collective actions. Unsurprisingly, the city-level Cyberspace Administration censored this online patient alliance group, which was then reported to the local health authority, and informed the district-level government and party committees as well. The potential collective action has become a priority for the local cadres to deal with during the critical political time.

The medical mediation committee took the lead and one of the most experienced mediators was soon called and dispatched to resolve this emergency case. There formed a headquarter centered in medical mediation committee, while keeping the local police authority, health bureau, as well as the party secretary of the district in the report line. The mediator said.

> Before retirement, I was the police officer and now was recruited as the part-time mediator. I received the call from the mediation committee at weekend and soon went to Zhejiang province (the group leader's home) quickly with three hours' drive from the city. I am not alone, and was accompanied by the local police and neighborhood representatives. He was apparently shocked by my presence at his home and told me that he has done nothing wrong.[9]

Mr. X was apparently shocked by this visit. Although he has experience in petitioning the local government, it is his first time organizing a cross-province collective action, which renders higher political risks (Chen & Yang, 2023). From his understanding, their target is a private hospital rather than a public one and did not involve anything political and the collective action has never taken place yet. And their action is also morally justified since they are all "deceived" by the hospital. The mediator took a various serious tone, and said "unreported and unapproved public assembly was a very serious violation of the law, and you know that. Next week, the entire society is expecting the first plenary session of the Central Committee of the Communist Party of China. What is your objective for organizing this?"[10] Mr. X was surely felt shocked of this severe "accusation" as the mediator framed their cross-regional activities as lodging the protest against the government, which he did not intend to. He soon surrendered and clarified that he was satisfactory with the government, and just want to punish the private hospital for stealing money from their people who was already miserable and vulnerable. He soon texted the whole online group to cancel the visit and refund the money to the petitioners. To prevent the resurgence, one police officer also joined the online group as an undercover agent to monitor the online chat room in order to report to the mediator whenever necessary and identify the leader or active members of the group. A potential collective action was resolved before it could have taken place.

Many patients use collective actions to vent their dissatisfaction towards the health institutions. Their vulnerable and powerless identity often provided the justification for their disruptive actions by winning the sympathy of the public. The mediators

---

[9] Author's interview with mediator H, October 2017.

[10] Author's interview with mediator H, October 2017.

highlighted the importance of a politicization strategy to make patients be aware of the sensitivity of the dispute by considering the larger picture of social stability. By framing their disruptive actions as an attempted politicized incident as an approach of political persuasion, it delegitimizes the disputants and constrains the occurrence of social disturbances.

It might be difficult for others to understand how the mediation and persuasion work is conducted by merely the mediators as half laymen. In fact, in the mediation process, the mediators did not work alone. They often worked with various bureaus including police officers in cases that involve potential collective actions that might have endangered social stability or during critical times. For instance, in the case discussed above, it is a well-coordinated stability maintenance activity composed of multiple departments across regional borders. The periphery actors, including local neighborhood committees and local police offices where the activist resided, the health bureau in the target city, etc. It involved the collaboration with various government departments as well as cross-province co-ordination, under the facilitation of the mediation committees. By doing so, the mediation committee could not only redirect the patients from collective actions to their channel but also satisfy the local government's stability maintenance concerns through adopting flexible measures.

Since the medical dispute mediation committee received funding and subsidy from the government as the government purchasing service, they have the natural inclination to spare the government burden. Preventing and dissolving collective action has become the major yet fundamental requirement and criteria in measuring the mediators' performance. The mediation committee often proactively identifies the potential risks and keeps each department posted, working with various government bureaus horizontally, in order to demonstrate the competency of the mediation committees. In the case discussed, in the fieldwork city, the mediation committee has developed a standard protocol to deal with cases that might involve collective actions. The mediation committees would report to and collaborate with police, juridical bureau, as well as keep vice district-level cadre noticed upon identifying politically sensitive disputes or those that might attract unwanted public or media attention. The internal briefing system has been well established to avoid the occurrence and escalation of collective action through drawing various government departments together. In return, the supervisory local juridical office would highly praise the mediators who prevent cases of collective actions by granting various honorable positions. For instance, the mediator who successfully prevented the collective action during the sensitive timing received the award of the outstanding mediator that year. The honorary award also motivated mediators to work harder to intervene the medical dispute resolution and act as role models for other mediators.

Meanwhile, mediators would be more incentivized to check disputants' behaviors and identify the potential risks of collective actions during certain national or critical events. According to the policy on people's mediation in Ningxia, each district/county must report potential disputes to the higher-level government on a monthly basis. However, during especially sensitive periods, all relevant parties, including mediation committees, are required to report on a daily basis to resolve disputes efficiently.[11] For instance, the patient Zhou in Heze City, Shandong province, got an emergency hysterectomy after she lost her unborn baby. She threatened to petition Beijing during the 19th Congress meeting, which also attracted the local official's attention. Local people's congress representative and local cadre all intervened.[12] Their intervention prevented the potential skip-level petition from taking place. The mediators shared with pride that they successfully averted a collective action against one public hospital because such collective actions would not only endanger stability but also generate health risks associated with public gatherings during the Covid-19 pandemic.[13]

Politicizing strategy is often applied to deter the potential activists to maintain the social stability flexibility without resorting to force. In prior, mediators intervened after the collective actions or petitioning took place. Today, as a result of the comprehensive stability maintenance mechanism, the mediation channel has been incorporated into the system, and the goals of the mediators is to prevent the occurrence of the collective actions. They usually employ the politicizing tactic to draw the red line between what is acceptable from the government, and which is not, as the "messenger" from the government to deter the collective actions. The timing of the disputes is also critical to explaining the mediators' proactive response. For these types of cases that took place at critical moment or involve collective actions, the mediators often paid with extra time and patience, to contain the political risk.

4.3.3 *Affective Strategy*

In addition to the politicization approach, the affective strategy is the most frequent and effective way to persuade the disputants in the mediation process. As discussed, mediators enjoyed high social status in the community. The mediators shoulder the responsibility not only to "find the justice" for the disputants, but also to win their trust and provide necessary social and emotional assistance to the disputants to untie their knot in the heart, which is believed as the major difference between mediation and other channels in dispute resolution. According to Hu Jieren et al.'s study (Hu et al., 2018), the mediation frequently performs the role of the emotion labor or social worker to provide a good level of psychological comfort, which lessen citizen's inclination to resort to collective action or continue the lawsuit. It better satisfies the political goal of "source management" by relieving the anger and grievance and winning their trust from the bottom of the disputants' hearts. In practice, professional mediators also are encouraged to have a professional background in social work and

---

[11] See, for instance, People's Government of Ningxia Hui Autonomous Region, Opinion on Further Strengthening the Mediation Work, https://www.nx.gov.cn/zwxx_11337/zwdt/202104/t20210425_2797852.html, accessed on May 18, 2024; author's interview with an officer from the judicial authority, on September 19, 2017.

[12] See, for instance, Disputes arising from medical accidents, representatives help to resolve, http://www.hezerd.gov.cn/view.asp?id=10424&classid=48, accessed on September 30, 2023.

[13] Author's follow-up interview with mediator, August 2020.

practical experience in psychology or seniority in age to better exhibit sympathy and compassion and establish personal connections (guanxi) with the disputants. Hence, many of the full-time mediators are social workers, and their role is to make friends and exchange hearts with the disputants, which are believed to efficiently reduce conflict sensitivity and the risk of confrontation.

Mediators believed that politicization strategy could only deter the disputant by "coercive force" temporarily, the affective strategy was the final and most effective cure for the disputants. For example, in the above-mentioned case of the planned collective action by patients of ankylosing spondylitis, after the leader of the online patient alliance gave up his plan for cross-regional activism, the mediator soon softened his tone and showed how he sympathized the patients' misfortune and status. The mediator promised the group leader Mr. X that they could count on him that he would represent the whole affected patient group to talk to the private hospital, which could be more effective than their activities. The mediator told the author that,

> The patients involved are very miserable. Many of them are disabled and the leader also has difficulties walking. They used to think that the treatment could cure the disease, while it is not true as the disease is incurable. I do feel pity for them. But you can also imagine, in such as critical political timing, a large group of disabled people gathered in front of the private hospital (which is located close to the business center and the airport). It would attract much-unwanted attention and unfaithful report on social media. This is something we need to prevent and could not afford. But as long as they choose our mediation channel, we would give priority to their case. At the same time, we also need to show our empathy to the patients. It is a humane way to do so.[14]

For the majority of disputants, regardless of their social and economic status, the common characteristic is heightened emotion, such as grievance, regret, and anger. Affective approach could efficiently comfort the disputants and reshape their behaviors. On the one hand, the mediators need to proactively display their positive emotions towards the disputants, such as support, relieve and trust. Many mediators commented that most of their work is beyond working hours. For instance, some commonly applied affective tactics of mediators include sending holiday greeting messages, casual chatting frequently with disputants and their family members, sharing personal stories with disputants to build trust, etc. These works are often performed in mediators' leisure time, which are "unmeasurable" or hard to document. On the other hand, the mediators are also motivated to help generate insider information about the disputants to smooth the dispute resolution process. For instance, when mediators communicate with the patients, they would often give them hot water, and invite them to take a seat to show the friend gesture with the disputants. The key goal of the affective strategy is not only to make friends with disputants but to find their "real" demands, and gather the required information and understand their expectations for the mediation. Showing empathy towards the disputants is an effective way to shorten the distance between the mediators and disputants to open the disputant's heart. Some mediators commented that compared to the courts, the mediation channels are more humane. For instance, one mediator said,

[14] Author's interview with mediator H, October 2017.

> Once you showed enough empathy with the disputants, they would open their hearts and tell you what their biggest concerns are. But it also costs long hours of work. For instance, one miserable nonlocal family lost their child in the hospital and showed great grievance. I cuddled them and helped them process a lot of administration work at the hospital as they were illiterate and unfamiliar with the hospital administration. They shared their life experiences with me, they had already lost their daughter before, and their age made it hard for them to have another child. Knowing the difficulties of the disputants is very important, which helps me to evaluate the sensitivity of the case and apply discretional power when necessary. If you cannot grasp the whole story and the background of the disputant, it is hard to untie their knotting heart.[15]

Usually, the mediators carefully avoid confronting the disputants by discussing their case directly the first time since it would easily arouse their anger and cautiousness, or even suspicious attitude towards the mediators. As said by one mediator, "At first, the patient often has the wrong impression that we (mediators) are negotiating with them on behalf of the hospital, which often leads to distrust. So, you must make very clear you are the third party and would try every effort to help the patients settle the case."[16] In the medical dispute mediation process, the facts are not always straightforward as it involve professional knowledge and judgmental calls from medical professionals. Hence, the mediators must need to deal with caution. They often tried their efforts to provide other solutions rather than answering the key query to pacify the disputants. During the fieldwork, I found that some female mediators usually start by discussing domestic matters to make friends with the disputants. One female mediator commented,

> Communication is very important. As a female, I can easily sense the changing attitudes of the disputants, which helped me to evaluate whether they could accept the mediation plan I offered. As a female and a mother as well, my background could better resonate with the disputants, and I am very patient to hear what the disputants say. Through heartful exchange, the ice-breaking process was shortened which accelerated the dispute reconciliation process.[17]

While for the male mediators, different approaches are applied. They usually try to establish authority over the mediators to seek their compliance and reliance. For instance, one mediator used to be a police officer before retirement which helped him to win the complete trust of the disputants. He told the disputants that he is well acquaintance with the hospital representatives. For instance, in the case of the losing child of the nonlocal family, he told the parents that "Do not worry. The doctors are quite familiar with me. Before I became a mediator, I was a police officer and was often dispatched to that hospital to address disruptive cases there. They would 'give me face' and take my words."[18] Winning the trust and building authority of the disputants would empower the mediators to act on their behalf and solicit the disputants' compliance. The disputant was appreciative of mediator's efforts after the mediation, "I was touched by the mediator who communicated with me proactively

---

[15] Fieldwork in the representative of one mediation committee in July 2017.

[16] Interview with the one mediator with social worker background in August 2017.

[17] Fieldwork in the representative of one mediation committee in July 2017.

[18] Author's interview with mediator H, October 2017.

and visited me often during the mediation process. He helped me to fulfil all the procedural work. Without him, nothing could be achieved as we do not have any social connections in the city. He not only addressed the dispute, but also encouraged our family to live on."[19]

In the city, the average age of mediators is approximately 54 years old; their seniority in age is often a great asset when communicating with patients and families as they are believed more experienced and reliable. For the families from lower social class, mediators enjoyed a relative favorable position as they are in higher social status and wider connections. The status and power asymmetry shaped the dependent relations between mediator and disputants as the latter depend on the former to address their grievances. In the mediation process, the disputants often "count on" and rely on the mediators to bargain for themselves to find justice.

In fact, most citizens involved in the mediation channel are from socially vulnerable groups; 61.2 per cent of the patients in this study's sample were non-local residents who seek health services from other regions.[20] It often means the patients bear heavier economic burden as the lower health reimbursement rates and have severe and complex health conditions. The mediation process is free of charge, which satisfies the economic demands of patients. Mediators, being embedded within the political system, are much more resourceful than disputants. Socially disadvantaged groups rely on the specialty mediation channel to solve disputes on their behalf or use their word "to uphold justice for them" (zhuchi gongdao). Some of them often sent the pennant and thank-you letter to show how they appreciate the mediators' work to help them find justice. However, mediators are less effective at applying affective strategy to better-resourced disputants, with whom they struggle to establish personal trust and authority.

Of course, the affective strategy has different outcomes and not always successful. It is not always easy to build personal connections with the disputants. As one mediator remarked "it is much easier to establish authority over peasant farmers".[21] While in comparison, some of the disputants are from well-educated or middle-class families, and less responsive to the affective strategy. The other mediator commented,

> Some disputants, especially those intellectual ones, their attitudes are fine, but they are too stubborn and stick to their original plan. By comparison, as you know, peasants are very angry at first, but later, after my explanation, they will always calm down and accept my mediation plan. But for intellectuals, their attitudes are fine, but they just do not accept any plan.[22]

For instance, in April 2016, a third-tier hospital performed surgery on Miss G, a local resident in her early 20 s who had been diagnosed with a malignant brain tumour. Sadly, Miss G's condition deteriorated after the procedure. Her mother believed that

---

[19] Author's interview with a patient in August 2017.

[20] Author's interview with an officer from the judicial authority, September 19, 2017. The internal archival documents and case files covered the medical disputes mediation disputes from 2010 to 2017 in fieldwork city.

[21] Author's interview with mediator H, October 2017.

[22] Author's interview with mediator Y, September 2016.

the hospital should be held partially accountable for her daughter's suffering. The mediators informed the mother that the developing tumour, not the surgery, was to blame for her daughter's blindness after speaking with medical professionals. She did not agree with the mediators' justifications and medical report. The mediator texted the mother repeatedly throughout the mediation process and wanted to speak with her; she politely declined and stressed that she would sue the hospitals. The mediator commented that "the more knowledge [education] they have, the harder it is to convince them".[23] The mother lost the first lawsuit as well as the second appeal. The mediator explained to the author that it is very challenging to convince patients, especially urban and well-educated citizens, who strongly believe in their own judgements as they do not trust the mediators. Mediators find it hard to win the trust of such disputants.

In this situation, the disputants enjoyed relatively equal power relations with the mediators. The introduction of the mediation did not help to boost the status of the disputants greatly. Since the disputants did not need a broker or other intermediary to approach the doctors or make conversation with the hospitals, it often made the mediation process more difficult and prolonged.

4.3.4 Compensation Bargaining

The key to politicization and affective strategy is to limit and prevent the disputants from any disruptive actions that might endanger the social security. While the compensation bargaining is the final step and the core of the mediation. Although some disputants declared that they want justice for the beloved ones, there is always a "price" beneath, hence I term these claims as "moral-economic" ones. The goal of the mediators is to re-channel the disputants from right-protection activities to the economic compensation bargaining process in order to neutralize their claims and divert their focus to the material interests embedded in the dispute resolution. It not only dampens the political sensitivity of medical disputes, but makes the dispute resolution process more controllable and flexible. For example, in the case of Mr. C we discussed before, he emphasized that the poor family's economic situation was long stressed by his son's long-term treatment. He asked the hospital to compensate for all the money that they spent in raising their child. It might be unacceptable to give a price tag on the patient and determine the value of the depth of their family members' grief, yet the compensation was framed as the only remedy they could receive as a comfort. The mediator justified that, we also feel sorry for the disputants, yet they also need to be aware that the damage has been caused already and the only thing they could get is economic compensation, which we would help them fight for.[24]

---

[23] Ibid.

[24] Author's interview with mediator H, October 2017.

In medical dispute resolution, the foremost issues are whether or not and how much one can receive as economic compensation. As discussed, the principal rationale in deciding the amount of compensation relies on the responsibility attribution after the medical examination. Today, to prevent the citizens' disruptive behaviors at the hospitals motivated by economic reasons, public hospitals are very cautious in compensating the patients at no fault. They often hired a team of professional lawyers in dealing with the lawsuits and cases through the mediation channel. As some mediators complained, "Nowadays, whenever there is a mediation meeting involving tertiary hospital, a bunch of lawyers would always line in front me, which also make me feel pressured".[25] As the hospital increasingly applies legal weapons to protect their rights, the compensation bargaining process is not easy.

The author has found one of the largest-ever compensation cases on record in the fieldwork city. During which, the mother filed a medical dispute over her eight-year-old son's accidental death. She and her husband sent their boy to the hospital in early morning when he complained of having a stomach-ache. In the early morning, it also happened to the be doctors on changing shift. In a rush, the doctor examined the boy, prescribed some pills and asked him to rest as the pain is not severe at that time. However, out of everyone's expectation, the poor boy's condition did not improve upon reaching home. In the 4 pm afternoon, he felt much worse, and the parents rushed him to the hospital again by taxi. Yet, the traffic congestion made the poor boy died on the way to the hospital.[26] The tragic loss devastated the family. The parents alleged that the doctor-in-charge did not consider their son's case as serious or emergency case because of their busy work shift, thus they filed to claim RMB3 million (US$454,500) in compensation.

Different from the prior practices which hospital often spending unnecessary compensation in exchange for peace, the tertiary hospital involved firmly protected their own interests. The hospital representative considered the mother's pursuit is irrational and blackmail as they insisted on the doctor's innocence. The mediation process was halted. The mediator persuaded the parents that, the hospital would not compensate them without adequate evidence as once they did, it would start an unpleasant precedent for the hospitals to compensate patients that they are not liable to. As discussed, any large compensation cases must proceed the medical examination and, in their case, the child need to have a post-mortem examination, which is hard to accept in the Chinese culture. The parents consulted one of their relative who was a nurse in one hospital, and finally agreed to perform the medical examination of their son to seek the truth of the boy's death and provide sufficient evidence for their case. After independent and third-party medical examination, it showed their son had died of intussusception, which could have been found and treated if the doctor had taken an X-ray or performed a CT (computed tomography) scan. It holds the hospital and the doctor liable as the latter misdiagnose the symptoms.

Now, the situation favored the disputants. According to the medical malpractice regulation, the hospital and doctor have the high possibilities of losing the case if the

[25] Based on author's fieldnote, interview with a mediator in September 2017.

[26] Based on author's fieldnote, October 2017.

mediation channeled to the lawsuits and the hospital as well as the doctors would receive the administrative penalty. To strike the balance, the mediators began to do the thought work for both sides. On the one hand, the mediator convinced the hospital to provide a higher compensation amount which is up to 1.8 million (US$278,700) and official apology from the hospitals. On the other hand, the mediator now again intervened to persuade the parents to stay in the mediation channel and not resort to legal channels. The mediator said,

> I have been following the case for a long time. After building the connection with the disputant, I find that the parents are very pitiable. But they should also be aware of that their son has already left, and there is nothing else they can make up except accepting the money. I told them that even if they file a lawsuit, according to the local guidance and regulation, usually the suggested compensation for the deceased is one million RMB as the ceiling, and they also need to take the expensive rate charge of lawyers into account. Yet, now the hospital offered more money in the mediation channel, and our mediation channel is free of charge. The compensation is higher than any prior precedents. I suggest them to take the money and move on with their life, which is difficult of course.[27]

The mediator persuaded the parents to be realistic and provided solid justification through relating to prior court cases as reference. To some extent, the mediator successfully not only keep the disputant stay in the mediation channel, but also reshape their demand and expectation to a great extent. Fearing prolonged lawsuits and repeated mentioning their sad past, the family agreed on the compensation offered by the mediators. The mediator continued, "after all, accept or not, the money could be the only remedy you can receive."[28]

Meanwhile, the mediators also proactively manage and reshape the disputants' perceptions and expectations towards the monetary compensation. When the disputant visited the mediation committee for the first time, the mediator would record their desired amount of the compensation. It sometimes becomes an important key performance indicator to measure the success of mediation by comparing the compensation gap between the before- and after-mediation. Using the mediators' term, the mediation process aimed to help the disputants to internalize the grievance, and also make them be "reasonable" in asking for the compensation. They would provide the disputants with solid and professional legal information to make them for give up high expectations. For instance, the involved legal documents include the "Tort Liability Law", "X City Compensation Standards for Personal Injury", and the "Interpretation of the Supreme People's Court on Several Issues Concerning the Application of Law in the Trial of Personal Injury Compensation Cases". Through law popularization, it aimed to manage the disputants' expectations to decrease their monetary claims.

When the above regular measures failed, the mediators would also strategically apply the "psychological warfare" to influence patients' attitudes, decisions, and behaviors covertly. One common tactic of the mediators is to manage the expectations of the disputants through the *delaying strategy*. As the disputants are always urgent

---

[27] Author's interview with mediator W, September 2017.

[28] Ibid.

to address their grievances, any delay in the process would make them feel anxious and fatigued. The mediators are experienced in controlling the changing mindsets and attitudes of the disputants. Through the delaying tactic, it often succeeded in persuading the disputants to take a lower settlement or compensation offer to end the long process. For instance, one mediator shared her experience:

> When the patient comes to the mediation committee, they often have some unrealistic expectations as many lawyers often brainwash them to pursue a large number of compensation to make money. When you find their claims are so high that there is no way the hospital could address them and the patients are hard to persuade, you could leave the patient alone for a longer time, such as a cooling-off period. Then, they would be aware of the fact that if he insisted on the original amount, he might end up receiving not one penny. We (mediators) would also not spoil them by satisfying their non-pragmatic claims. Then, after this period, he would usually come back to you, and we can reassume the dialogue. This re-connecting with the patient would make the patients accept lower compensation.[29]

In addition to managing the disputant's attitudes by controlling the pace of the mediation, the mediators also apply precedent case as evidence to help the disputants lower their expectations. The principle of the compensation distribution is elusive, and largely based on the mediators' own understanding and judgements. The experienced mediators consciously promoted the consistent compensation distribution by stipulating the creation of the pool of reference cases and making decisions based on the precedents. Only when disputants corroborate their arguments by providing more evidence can they break the precedents. Patients must provide adequate proof or seek a third-party medical examination and other justifications to increase their bargaining power in the compensation distribution. One mediator said that,

> After years of experience, we can tell whether the compensation is reasonable based on past cases. If you break the precedent one time, later, it will put you in a difficult situation and hard to convince the disputants in the future.[30]

By doing so, it gradually formed a consistent pattern and norm in compensating the disputants which largely lowered their expectations towards the compensation. Different from the tactic of satisfying the patients' demands at all costs, mediators also perform as legal half-layman to uphold the law to avoid overcompensating. For instance, according to a case that occurred in another city, the family claimed that the medical tragedy not only made them lose their daughter but also cost them economic gains (at least 50 square meters of apartment) in the recent house demolition activity. They requested the hospital also make compensation for their economic loss in the demolition process, which included buying a three-room apartment for the deceased and the hospital representative needed to in present on every tomb sweeping day to show their remorse, etc. Despite the disruptive strategies the patients have adopted, the mediators uphold the standard strictly and repeatedly persuade the disputant to follow the law and regulation. The involved mediators noted, "the disputant once said he would accept the offer as long as the hospital could add a few more thousand

---

[29] Interview with Mediator W, September 2017.

[30] Author's field notes, interviews with mediators in several districts, August to September 2017.

RMB, but I refuse. I repetitively told the disputant that we are the third-party and should be objective."[31] At last, the disputant accepted the original offer suggested by the mediator and made a formal apology for the disruptive actions. During the mediation process, the mediators did not bow to the pressure made by the disputants. Sometimes, the disputant makes extreme demands, and mediators would selectively make a concession, yet be cautious to not bow to every aggressive move from the disputant. Once the disputant finds distributive processes are negotiable, it could push the mediators to the corner. Hence, mediators vigorously protect the bottom line in distributive negotiations to ascertain their neutral organization-al identity and organizational trust.

It is also necessary to admit that the mediators also apply discretional occasionally. Given the flexibility of the mediation committees, mediators are often provided with discretional power in compensation distribution. It could be flexibly applied to disputants that warrant special attention by breaking the precedent. For instance, one chief representative of the mediation committee told the author that there used to be non-local woman in her early 40s experienced miscarriage after receiving the third assisted reproduction therapy. The hospital interpreted the miscarriage as nature and beyond the boundary of the malpractice, while the mediator told the hospital representative to do a favor considering the miserable situation of the women. The mediator said,

> The surgery cost her a lot of money, and it was her third miscarriage, which the husband blamed her a lot. She accidentally caught a cold when arriving the city. The doctor said it did not matter and performed the surgery. That's why she blamed the doctor for this. Doctors are not liable for this, but I convinced the hospital to compensate the women by reimbursing the treatment fee to maintain the harmonious relations with patients.[32]

In China, the previous long-lasting one-child policy gave children a central role in the family and made them the binding glue of various social relations. An innocent child patient involved in a medical dispute attracts the attention of families, society, and the media. When addressing cases involving children, mediators are careful to prevent the cases from escalating to social discontent by strengthening the political importance of solving disputes.

As the liaison between the hospital and patients, the mediators enjoyed the discursive power not only to persuade the patients but also the hospitals. In cases that involve vulnerable patients or cases that have great potential that might lead to collective actions, the mediators would take the initiative and convince the hospitals to higher compensation. Mediation sometimes persuades hospitals to consider not only the medical facts but also the political concern, such as avoiding social conflict, and the moral concern, such as showing empathy to disadvantaged social groups by strengthening the political importance of maintaining social stability. From the mediator's perspective, offering monetary compensation did not hamper the authority

[31] Based on author's fieldwork. See, also Mediation case of medical dispute between Wang's family and a hospital in Beijing, http://alk.12348.gov.cn/Detail?dbID=48&dbName=RTHZ&sysID=25, accessed on September 30, 2023.

[32] Author's interview with mediator X, August 2016.

of the mediation, but it enabled some patients to show gratefulness to the institutions upon recognizing that the mediators have broken the precedents for them. It also greatly discourages them from applying disruptive actions in hospitals. From the hospital perspective, it is often cost-efficient to avoid prolonged lawsuits and unwanted disruptive actions in the public space. Hospitals are also willing to "give a face" (provide favor) to the mediator's suggestions occasionally since they all belong to the component of the synthesized social stability maintenance chain to maintain order in hospitals.

Taken together, mediators are experienced to adopt delaying tactics to avoid direct confrontation with the patients as well as to exert psychological pressure on the disputants to lower their expectations towards monetary bargaining. Meanwhile, they are also sophisticated in persuading the disputants by referring to precedent to enhance the institutional authority and consistency of their decisions. Thirdly, the mediators also apply discretional power to make exceptions to pitiable patients or difficult cases that warrant more flexibility.

4.4 Summary

As the quote from Han Feizi said, "Following the patterns (li) of the heavens, then things could be achieved without effort (Chen, 2000)." The mediators followed the procedures and developed a series of strategies to redress the disputes and unknot the patient's heart. This chapter demonstrates the daily practice of the mediators in the medical dispute mediation process. Mediation channels could prevent the occurrence of collective actions which may endanger the stability maintenance, and be flexible in responding to the particular needs of the disputations without endangering the authority of the legal authorities; as well as being responsiveness to the emotional demands of the disputants. This chapter detailed the three strategies commonly applied by the mediators—politicization, affective and economic bargaining—that not only contribute to stability maintenance goals but also satisfy psychological needs and promote consistent decisions. In detail, they utilize the politicization strategy to deter disputants and prevent and counter collective actions by working horizontally with relevant government authorities. Affective strategy aims to build personal trust with disputants, improve and develop personal ties to smoothen the mediation process, acquire information, and alleviate personal grievances. Economic bargaining strategy aims to shift citizens' attention from rights protection towards compensation to neutralize their claims, and to strengthen institutional authority by using precedents to shape patients' expectations.

The passage of the People's Mediation Law in 2010 has brought about profound changes in mediation institutions, which has led to the specialization of the mediation committees. The mediation committee has not only become effective in dispute resolution, but also gradually gained professionalism and formalism. By promoting the mediation channel in addressing wicked problems in the C city since 2010, the mediation committees have become prevalent across China. From the government's perspective, the increasing number of civil disputes, which are often accompanied by disruptive actions, has posed new challenges for the maintenance of grassroots stability. The essential components of dispute resolution can be met by developing an institutional channel to resolve disputes and absorb social grievances. As a result, the judicial department, together with the professional management units, can guide and monitor specialty mediation committees to provide profession-based advice and to maintain social stability by utilizing and centralizing all resources. More importantly, specialty mediation committees are also becoming more professional by focusing on only one type of dispute and adhering to precedents, which strengthen their authority and promote consistent decisions.

Experienced mediators and their political- and social- embeddedness are the key to success. Their existence not only helped to address the social dispute "on behalf of" the local government, but also resembles the social gentry in the old days that worked in the third realm, as an intermediary to connect grassroots personnel and public institutions. Through their intermediary role, they better break the power asymmetry and are responsive towards the moral-economic claims raised by the vulnerable (Huang, 1993). As discussed, there exists a power asymmetry between the patients and hospital representatives, and such injustice in social power is often reproduced in the medical dispute resolution process, which carries the possibility of leading to disruptive actions. The introduction of government-embedded mediators rewrote the relations. Mediators contribute to granting the disputants access to resources, boosting the patients' bargaining power, and promoting a fair tie between the disputants and hospitals. They are the active agents in the process, rather than passively implementing the government decisions. These strategies not only shape the disputants' mindsets but also project positive views of the mediation channels and enhance institutional authority and professionalism. Their seniority, authority, and political embeddedness allow them to negotiate between hospitals and patients in dispute resolution. Applying coercion and soft persuasion interchangeably, contributed to the tranquility in the society and the high-resolution rate.

Power continues to be embedded in and shape the development and process of medical dispute mediation. The mediation process facilitated was full of power interactions. On the one hand, the source of mediators' authority was their seniority in terms of social status and their political status embedded in the Mediation Committee. By establishing authority over the patients and doctors, the mediators sought compliance and trust during the mediation process and could influence the mediation outcome. On the other hand, the element of guanxi (connections) may also play an important role in shaping the results of mediation. The political background and connections of the Mediation Committee allowed mediators to intervene and seek compliance from the patients and doctors when there was an imbalance between them. For patients, having more guanxi through personal and organizational ties could push the hospitals to take them seriously, possibly giving them a more favorable position in the bargaining process. Establishing the authority of the mediating institution may help patients resolve medical disputes in a balanced power structure. It aims to make patients feel like they are on equal footing with doctors and hospitals, facilitating the dispute resolution and increasing the personal efficacy in the resolution process.

The mediation is not flawless. Chinese governors should also consider institutionalizing the mediation system by promoting a more transparent information flow and introducing a third-party evaluation system to better protect the rights of both patients and hospitals. Doctors and patients may feel invisible pressure during the mediation process and need to address incomparable top-down bureaucratic and political power. Separating politics from medicine could better help structure the mediation process and protect the rights of patients and hospitals. Second, this study finds that laypersons may be biased towards the plaintiffs (patient) when addressing medical disputes (Liang, 2003). Mediators, though enjoying seniority and a recognized status in society, may not be capable of dealing with professional medical cases. Moreover, the current institutional design is not prepared to take on high caseloads. One mediator could not track very many cases at the same time. This system demonstrates the use of power to influence and promote agreement achievement between patients and hospitals through authority, by controlling the information flow, and using coercive means and sanctions. This system recreates a new power dynamic among the key stakeholders and overcomes the power imbalance among patients and hospitals.

The mediation process is still biased, and result-oriented, and the efficiency of dispute resolution may still rely on the disputants' negotiating power and characteristics. As the fieldwork shows, the efficacy of the mediation channel varied among the various socio- and economic- statuses of the disputants. Mediation institutions may be more effective at persuading vulnerable groups that lack formal legal assistance, time, and resources. In contrast, for instance, for the cases that involve intellectuals, as disputants' relatively equal power relations the mediators find it harder to establish authority over the urban middle class.

Furthermore, by placing greater weight on social stability and preventing the occurrence of bottom-up collective actions, the mediation process tends to only accept top-down fine-tuning and lacks the motivation to promote systematic and institutional change. The mediators are also under constant pressure to settle the compensation claims in an efficient manner. How do mediators distribute compensation to medical disputes to balance various goals at the same time? In the next chapter, the author will empirically investigate the outcome of the mediation to further unveil the dark box of the mediation and how the patient and hospital shaped the mediation outcomes jointly through compensation bargaining.

References

Baldwin, D. A. (1978) Power and social exchange. *American Political Science Review, 72*(4): 1229–1242.

Bian, Y. (1994) Guanxi and the allocation of urban jobs in China. *The China Quarterly, 140*: 971–999.

Blau, P. (2017) *Exchange and power in social life*: Routledge, New York.

Carlson, T. N. (2019) Through the grapevine: Informational consequences of interpersonal political communication. *American Political Science Review, 113*(2): 325–339.

Chen, X., & Yang, K. (2023) The Puzzle of Cross-Provincial Activism in China: From Relational Dynamics to State Strategies: From Relational Dynamics to State Strategies. *Comparative Politics, 55*(4): 597–615.

Chen, Qiyou. 2000. "Han Fei Zi xin jiaozhu" ("Han Feizi, with new collations and com-mentary") (Shanghai Classics Publishing House).

Dahl, R. A. (1957) The concept of power. *Behavioral science, 2*(3): 201–215.

Granovetter, M. (2018) Economic action and social structure: The problem of embeddedness. In *The sociology of economic life* (pp. 22–45) Routledge.

Hu, J., Wu, T., & Fei, J. (2018) Flexible governance in China: Affective care, petition social workers, and multi-pronged means of dispute resolution. *Asian Survey, 58*(4): 679–703.

Huang, P. C. (1993). "Public Sphere"/" Civil Society" in China? The Third Realm between State and Society. *Modern China, 19*(2): 216–240.

Huang, P. C. (2006) Court mediation in China, past and present. *Modern China, 32*(3): 275–314.

Hwang, K. K. (1987) Face and favor: The Chinese power game. *American journal of Sociology, 92*(4): 944–974.

Jasper, J. M. (2011) Emotions and social movements: Twenty years of theory and research. *Annual review of sociology, 37*: 285–303.

Jasper, J. (2004) A strategic approach to collective action: Looking for agency in social-movement choices. *Mobilization: An International Quarterly, 9*(1): 1–16.

Liang, B. A. (2003) Layperson and physician perceptions of the malpractice system: implications for patient safety. *Social science & medicine, 57*(1): 147–153.

Liebman, B. L. (2013) Malpractice mobs: medical dispute resolution in China. *Columbia Law Review*: 181–264.

Lukes, S. (1974) *Power: A Radical View*. Palgrave Macmillan.

Martin, J. L. (2002) Power, authority, and the constraint of belief systems. *American Journal of Sociology, 107*(4): 861–904.

Michelson, E. (2007) Climbing the dispute pagoda: grievances and appeals to the official justice system in rural China. *American sociological review, 72*(3): 459–485.

Pye, M. W., & Pye, L. W. (2009) *Asian power and politics: The cultural dimensions of authority*. Harvard University Press.

Studdert, D. M., Mello, M. M., Gawande, A. A., Gandhi, T. K., Kachalia, A., Yoon, C., ... & Brennan, T. A. (2006) Claims, errors, and compensation payments in medical malpractice litigation. *New England journal of medicine, 354*(19): 2024–2033.

Wall Jr, J. A., & Blum, M. (1991) Community mediation in the People's Republic of China. *Journal of Conflict Resolution, 35*(1): 3–20.

Wilson, E. J., & Sherrell, D. L. (1993) Source effects in communication and persuasion research: A meta-analysis of effect size. *Journal of the academy of marketing science, 21*, 101–112.

Zhang, J., & Cai, Y. (2019) Medical disputes and mediation in China: Government and responsibility shifting. *China Information, 33*(3): 350–371.

Zhuang, W., & Chen, F. (2015) "Mediate First": The revival of mediation in labour dispute resolution in China. *The China Quarterly, 222*: 380–402.

Chapter 5
From Right Protection to Monetary Bargaining

Rationale in Compensation Distribution

无功者受奖，则财溃而民望。
If those who have no merit are rewarded, the fortunes will be ruined, and the popularity of the people will be lost.
—Han Feizi 韩非子《饰邪》*[On Pretensions and Evils]*
故至治之国，有赏罚而无喜怒。
In the most governed country, there are rewards and punishments but no joy or anger.
—Han Feizi 韩非子《用人》*[Employing People]*

In recent decades, Chinese government has frequently utilized the "buying stability" strategy as a compromise in exchange for the inactive of the disputants to maintain social stability and prevent the occurrence of collective actions (Lee & Zhang, 2013). However, buying stability is not always a perfect solution. The frequent appliance of buying stability has inevitably provided economic incentives and "encouraged" citizens to resort to troublemaking tactics to realize personal interests or prioritize their claims. It may also deteriorate government-citizen relationships in responding to the disputant's claims. Today, the government has gradually shifted the dispute resolution, and specifically, its compensation distribution responsibility to the third party—People's Mediation Committees. The mediation channel has further institutionalized the compensation distribution process through bargaining between patients and hospitals, giving rise to a series of unanswered questions: What's the embedded rationale in compensation distribution? How do the patients' and hospitals' attributes affect the compensation outcome? How does the people's mediation promote consistent compensation distribution?

In this Chapter, I aim to dive into investigating the rationale embedded in the compensation distribution to settle medical disputes, drawing on evidence from people's mediation committees of medical disputes. This chapter argues that the people's mediation committee has performed as a centralized bargaining channel to promote compensation distribution systematically to settle the dispute. Through

---

The earlier version of this Chapter is published by Jie Wu, "People's Mediation Committees: Bargaining Between Hospitals and Patients." Journal of Chinese Political Science 26, no. 2 (2021): 353–371 (Springer).

J. Wu, *Politicized Medical Dispute Resolution in China*, Understanding China,
https://doi.org/10.1007/978-981-97-6961-2_5

the mediation channel, the focus of the dispute resolution also shifted from rights discourse to responding the monetary compensation claims raised by the disputants, which also de-politicized the nature of the social disputes. By reviewing medical dispute case files empirically, I find that compensation outcomes may be influenced by a series of interactions of distributive justice, political stability reasons, and economic concerns. Through the mediation channel, the Chinese government could resort to a non-coercive and preventive approach to manage social disputes flexibly.

5.1 Money Matters: Bargained Authoritarianism

Scholarly interest in the occurrence of social disputes and diversified the government's responses in China is growing rapidly. Since the 1990s, to prioritize their demands, social groups including peasants, homeowners, veterans, etc. often take collective actions or disruptive actions that across the boundary of the legitimate channel (O'Brien & Li, 2006; Chen, 2012; Tsai, 2015), which were considered threats to society stability. To maintain social tranquility, the central government used the cadre responsibility system to motivate the local government to prevent the occurrence the social disturbances and unrest. Under the pressure of "veto power",[1] local officials sometimes apply repression and extra-legal measures to discipline the activists and address disputes. However, it is not always the whole story.

Although coercive institutions have been crucial in any regimes to maintain social and political stability, the government did not always apply coercive or violent means. In fact, nowadays, the government increasingly applies non-coercive strategies in exchange for peace, such as censorship, information control, etc. (Davenport, 2005; 2007; Earl, 2003, 2004, 2011; Noakes & Gillham, 2007). In Putin's Russia, for instance, instead of resorting to violence, the government applied pre-emptive strategies such as surveillance and digital censorship against activists to prevent the occurrence of social unrests (Yusupova, 2022). It is all perceived as distinctive from violent repression but invisibly discourages citizens from undertaking collective actions by increasing their participation cost.

In China, the local governments are also aware that the frequent appliance of repression could also backfire or endanger legitimacy. Hence, in addition to the "sticks", in practice, "carrots" are also frequently applied in exchange for social stability at lower political cost (Benney, 2016; Lee & Zhang, 2013; Zhuang & Chen, 2015). It is considered more cost-efficient, and more desirable than applying coercion directly to address the social unrests (McCarthy, Britt, and Wolfson, 1991; Earl, 2003; Davenport, 2007). This chapter adds a new line to this line of study by illustrating the

[1] Veto power leads cadres to be accountable to the hard and soft targets set by the higher government. See, for instance, Edin 2003.

application of buying stability as an alternative to governing the society while maintaining the regime's legitimacy, as well as examining its rationale in compensation distribution.

Buying stability (花钱买平安) refers to the institutions' efforts to redistribute public goods or provide monetary incentives to seek popular support and discourage potential social unrests under political pressure. For instance, Amengual (2018) studied the redistribution of compensation in Bolivia. Private firms apply strategies to selectively distribute benefits and public goods to people in exchange for stability. In China, however, monetary compensation distribution in response to social disputes remains state-centric. To ensure social stability and prevent the escalation of disputes, the government sometimes provides monetary benefits to the targeted individuals or social groups to address the dispute. For instance, in rural China, Jonathan Benney (2016) observed that local officials would occasionally distribute petty money to troublemakers to prevent their skip-level petitioning activities at politically sensitive moments. It also has become a common practice in dispute or protest bargaining by distributing monetary benefits to the leaders as a divide-and-conquer strategy to discourage collective actions.

Lee Ching Kwan and Zhang Yonghong (2013) summarized this practice as bargained authoritarianism:

> These processes allow aggrieved citizens a certain degree of political leverage and relatively expansive opportunities to obtain material concessions and symbolic rewards from the state (p. 1503–1504).

The increasing utilization of buying stability, though demobilized and divided the activities successfully and efficiently at critical moments, has also led to unexpected outcomes. Although bargained authoritarian de-politicized the nature of the collective actions and contained the collective actions temporarily, it also commodified state-society relations embedded accompanied by the informal and illegitimate economic exchanges between state agents and citizens. Meanwhile, maintaining social stability through buying stability often involves heavy economic costs, which is hard to sustain in a longer time frame. More crucially, the frequent utilization of buying stability provided incentives for the citizens to apply disruptive actions for economic benefits. From the citizens' perceptive, buying stability was often perceived as a form of concession and tolerance from the government. The utilization of the buying stability strategy has increased the citizens' positive efficacy in applying disruptive actions to prioritize their claims. The political space of bargaining outside the formal institutions has therefore emerged.

Hence, the government has encountered a dilemma in applying the buying stability strategy: it is obvious that government authorities have strong incentives to discourage and contain the occurrence of collective actions through buying stability, while they also carefully avoid over-compensating the activists which would encourage activists to apply disruptive action for benefits by exposing the vulnerabilities of bargained authoritarianism, as well as adding heavy economic burden on the local government. In other words, the government has been trapped in the dilemma of making constant tradeoffs between economic and political stability concerns.

Under the conflicting motivations, inconsistent results have been found in the government compensating practices in utilizing buying stability tactics to address social disputes. On the one hand, the government tends to favor the groups or organizational interests for economic reasons. For instance, in addressing labor disputes, local governments are under strong motivations to perverse local industries and enhance local economic development by neglecting or partially satisfying the compensation requests of the workers. However, in response to unpaid wages, when employers failed to pay (already very low) wages, on which many workers rely for their daily survival, collective actions are often easily triggered (Su & He, 2010), and the scales would be tilted oppositely. For example, the disputants sometimes even adopt the "suicide show" to arouse the officials' attention and prioritize their claims (Fu, 2017). Citizens could also resort to collective actions or media strategy to increase the responsiveness of the government to prioritize their claims (Cai, 2005; Chen, 2009). The disruptive actions adopted by the activists could leverage their influence when negotiating with the government to hold it accountable. Under political pressure, local governments have to make concessions to collective actions and disruptive strategies. Local government needs to choose between group interests and individuals under either economic development or political stability pressure.

In China, addressing social disputes always involves a cost. In fact, in most cases, the core focus of dispute resolution lies in the final monetary settlement. Although buying stability has become a routinized approach in addressing disputes that involve collective actions and disruptive actions, the hidden mechanism of government-led compensation distribution remains mysterious and unclear. On the one hand, extant studies largely rely on the discrete cases to observe the compensation distribution practices across China, with a large variation. On the other hand, the underlined government motivations could be more complex than satisfying the stability maintenance goals. Over-responding to compensation may not only create financial burdens for the local government, but also augment the legitimacy crisis and encourage repetitive petitions driven by economic interests, which in return, may even endanger social stability. In China, I find that the government has gradually shifted the compensation distribution role to the people's mediation channel to avoid blame and promote consistent practices in exercising the tactic of buying stability in the 2010s. This Chapter, therefore, draws on the empirical case of medical disputes and systematically examines the principles underlying the importance of understanding the everyday practice of buying stability in dispute resolution. It contributes to the existing studies by examining the rationale embedded in bargained authoritarianism by providing empirical evidence.

Facing mounting demands based on personal grievances and compensation requests, the government has now delegated dispute resolution, particularly the compensation distribution responsibility, to the People's Mediation Committees. As such, People's Mediation, today, acted as the centralized bargaining channel to compensate the disputes. People's Mediation Committees have become as popular venues for individual disputants to address their disputes as well as pursue their monetary claims. They provide monetary settlements for all types of disputes ranging from compensation for divorce (Huang, 2005) to wages and pension bargaining in labor disputes (Zhuang & Chen, 2015; Hu, 2011). Through the mediation channel, the dispute resolution process has commodified into a bargaining process by applying material benefits to measure citizen's grievances or rights, as money becomes the solution to most disputes.

The advantage of patching mediation institutions up with bargaining functions is multi-folded. First, from the institutional perspective, mediation institutions therefore developed great complexity since the 2010s. The mediation channels have transformed from the old institutions to a new component of the social management system to address grievances and show governance accountability. Since the 2010s, the government has been particularly keen on promoting and refashioning the Maoist weapon to new aims. Mediation channels have been refashioned to be technology-driven and professional-based by incorporating professionals into the mediation team and adopting high-end technology, including blockchain, big data, artificial intelligence, etc. (Hu & Zhang 2023). The revitalization and increasingly crucial role of the mediation institutions has enhanced integrated social governance and overcome institutional inertia to allow timely responses to the changing state-society relations.

Second, for the government, it not only frees the government from being involved directly in dispute resolution but also detaches the government from the compensation distribution role. Direct involvement in the dispute resolution may often elicit the citizens' dissatisfactory towards the government. The government adopted the "agenda limitation" approach (Hinterleitner, 2017) to pass the responsibility as well as the "shift blame" to the professional mediation institutions as the new intermediary between disputant and public institutions or private organizations (Zhang & Cai, 2019). Since the mediation channel is sponsored by the government and staffed by semi-official personnel, the process and results of the compensation distribution are still politicized and reflect the government's interests in social stability. By shifting the compensation distribution goal to the mediation channel, the government could still reach its social governance goals by claiming credits from the mediation committees. As such, the establishment of the People's Mediation Committees has decreased the government's direct involvement in the civil dispute resolution process to free their hands without retreating from managing the private life of citizens, as well as disguising their direct responsibility for the outcomes of the compensation distribution and dispute resolution.

From the citizens' perspective, through the centralized bargaining channel, individuals can overcome the power and resource asymmetry between individuals and their counterparts and emerge in a more advantaged or equal position. For example, in labor disputes, the power asymmetry between workers and employers is the key concern and hinders dispute resolution. The revitalization of the Mediation Committee centralizes a bargaining channel that alters the power distribution among disputants. With the centralized bargaining channel, individual or group-based workers are expected to regain more equal positions in bargaining with their employers, which would facilitate the dispute resolution process.

Money becomes the central focus in the dispute resolution process, and the mediation channel becomes the crucial intermediary for the compensation distribution. In the case of medical disputes, the key to dispute resolution often lies in the amount of compensation awarded. For instance, to begin the mediation process, every dispute needs to propose a clear number of monetary claims raised by the patient. It is an essential component of the dispute resolution process for the two parties to agree on the amount of compensation, or to "rationalize" (helihua 合理化) their compensation claims through the efforts of mediators. The term "rationalization" refers to the usage of reasoning, political persuasion, and social authority to draw a reconciliation between the disputants, which usually results in a decrease in the amount of compensation. People's Mediation must strike a constant balance between patients and hospitals, mirroring the dilemma faced by rulers at all levels in China.

What's the rationale for the mediation institutions in distributing compensation? In other words, how buying stability strategy been refashioned and innovated under the mediation institutions? In this Chapter, new data was applied to answer the old question to illustrate the embedded logic under bargained authoritarianism. In the following section, I will first document and theorize the key elements in government-led compensation distribution by providing a new theoretical framework for analyzing the rationale of compensation distribution. Then, I will provide empirical evidence of mediation's patterns and outcomes in compensating the patients. In a nutshell, I find that the compensation distribution for dispute resolution is now under the dynamic interactions between political pressure of social stability, perception of justice, as well as economic concerns. The complex interactions between these factors shaped the consequences of the compensation distribution. The following section will provide both quantitative and qualitative evidence to examine the logic in compensation distribution in the people's mediation channel to settle disputes.

5.2 Rationale in Compensation Distribution

5.2.1 Framework of Rationale for Compensation Distribution

This study aims to provide a theoretical framework to understand the rationale for compensation distribution of people's mediation committees. I suggest that the outcomes of the compensation distribution to address social disputes are a function of three factors: (a) in the quest for distribution justice; (b) political stability maintenance concerns; and (c) economic cost concerns. The first factor was conceptualized as the legal positioning of the mediation committees. I argue that the people's mediation is situated between the legal and social institutions that not only follow the written rules and regulations but also need to satisfy the social perception of justice and social appropriateness by promoting distributive justice. The second factor theorizes the political objective of the mediation committees, which need to maintain social stability and prevent the occurrence of disruptions and collective actions. The third factor is conceptualized as the cost-efficient and bureaucracy's characteristics. As the economic cost increases, the mediation committees are less likely to adopt buying stability as a solution.

5.2.2 In Quest for Distributive Justice

People's mediations shoulder the responsibility of redressing the scales and holding justice for the masses. Then, what's the perception of justice from the mediation institutions' perspective? Some scholars find that the People's Mediation Committee performs a role similar to courts and other legal institutions in making judgments based on regulations and law in the quest for justice. For instance, Halegua's study (2008) showed that the mediation committee provides an alternative means for achieving substantive results similar to those that the formal (legal) system ought to produce (p. 321). Yet, in fact, in addition to laws and regulations, mediators must also consider social norms and social appropriateness to satisfy morality and social expectations and find justice for the disputants or use the official term "reason" (*li*). For instance, according to Article 21 in the People's Mediation Law, the mediators would adhere to the principle, have a good understanding of law and reason (*li*), and find justice for the disputants (mingfa xili, zhuchi gongdao).

The term "*li*", refers to the "reasonable order" as the basic philosophical notions of Confucianism (Siminota, 2020, p.108), reflecting the sound and coherent order of the society, state, and culture. The *li*-consciousness was deeply based on the cultural understanding of justice, though it might be neither law-based nor rule-abided. Sometimes, there is tension between the li and the law. For instance, Tong (2014) finds that the Chinese villagers were subjectively mobilized by the moral consciousness which combines morality as well as pragmatism to petition the government. Their long-term vulnerability and deprived social status provided the moral justification for the villagers to correct the status quo by applying collective actions. However, as long as it satisfies the public perception of "*li*" as it protected the interests of the poor and weak or affirms the basic social values, it was often rendered appropriate from the social expectation and the public's moral imagination, though it might be not always based on the law. Hence, as President Xi noted, the mediation institutions need not only to make sure to follow the law, but also to persuade the disputants through reason to not only settle the case but also to repair the social relations.[2]

The public perception of justice in China is often shaped by the outcome they received from the process, as scholars categorized it as "distributive justice" (He & Feng, 2021; Feng & Cao, 2014; Gallagher and Wang, 2011). He and Feng (2021) explained that because of Chinese citizens' unfamiliarity with the legal system, they could not differentiate between procedural justice and outcomes as they could not feel control over the legal process. Chinese citizens are more result-oriented and widely use the outcomes as a crucial measurement of the effectiveness of the system. The public perception of justice is pragmatic, result-oriented, and focused on personal gain and efficacy in the system. People's Mediation, to some extent, augmented the result-oriented trend and promoted distributive justice to increase the public

[2] See, for instance, Strengthening mediation work in the new era to help build a safer China at a higher level, https://www.chinalaw.org.cn/portal/article/index/id/31184.html, accessed on October 2, 2023.

feeling of efficacy towards the mediation system. The mediators, though have accumulated experience in dispute resolution, are still laypersons in the legal field and their understanding of justice is far from perfect. Their primary role is not legal workers, but semi-government agents in dispute resolution. The underlined principle of the mediation channel is not only legal- or rule-based, but to increase the "secureness, happiness, and boost the sense of gain"[3] (安全感、幸福感、获得感) through the mediation institution. Therefore, distributing justice that based on the combination of reason and law was an important component of the daily practice of mediation. The role of the mediators is to increase social appropriateness, reinforce the public perception of distributive justice, and make disputants stay tuned in the mediation channels. To align with the social norms and reflect the proxy of reason, it is a common practice to distribute more benefits to the disputants who are pitiable or affirm the moral order.

To investigate the practice of reason in compensation distribution, I use the medical results for the justice principles shaping compensation distribution. According to the regulation, the range of the compensation is based on the severity of the medical results with a clear causality. People who face severe medical consequences (e.g., disability or death) are more likely to receive higher compensation than those involved in cases that are not associated with negative medical outcomes. Compensating cases associated with severe medical results satisfies the public demand for "eye-for-an-eye" justice. The mediation committee is under high public pressure to find the reason for the claimants who suffered from medical "failure" regardless of the responsible distribution of the hospitals or lack of medical malpractice evidence. Hence, we expect to find that: claimants are more likely to receive more monetary compensation if they experienced more severe medical outcomes.

5.2.3 *Political Stability—Discretion to Troublemakers*

In addition to demonstrating the quest for distributive justice or reflecting the role of "li" (social appropriateness and justice) in the compensation distribution process, the distribution outcomes are also shaped by the disruptive strategies and tactics adopted by the disputants. As Chen Xi's study (2009, 2012) finds, activists could apply troublemaking tactics to gain attention from higher levels of the government to accelerate the dispute resolution process. If the disputant claimants are perceived as troublemakers, they are more likely to receive concessions and greater monetary compensation in exchange for stability.

In the medical dispute mediation process, given their health condition, patients are self-ordered and less disruptive. However, from the individuals' perspective, since human time and efforts are the most widely appreciated resources available for collective actions (Edwards & McCarthy, 2004; Cunningham et al., 2017; Schock, 2013), their commitment of time and resources to the process would also contribute

[3] Ibid.

to the increased bargaining power of the disputants. For instance, Diana Fu's (2017) study on labor disputes shows that the individual workers who petitioned frequently could efficiently motivate the officials to respond and consider the individual seriously. Hence, in medical dispute resolution, persistent claimants are considered the tough disputants or even "troublemakers" for local officials in dealing with.

Meanwhile, mediators are also inclined to spare more effort for the persistent disputants. Mediators have the heavier burden of dealing with persistent disputants who are unlikely to give up. For the mediators, they are under pressure to settle the cases in an efficient and "safe" manner. Their working performance is measured by the average number of processing days required to address medical disputes, as well as the invisible pressure to maintain social stability. As the fieldwork shows, the preferred settlement for one medical dispute lasts within one month. If disputants are willing to spend time in the bargaining process, it signals their persistence and discontent with the outcome, which is likely to result in more responsiveness from the mediators under their informal evaluation pressure. Mediators thus are sophisticated to categorize sensitive and difficult cases by allocating more time and efforts. Hence, their priority is often given to these persistent claimants and claimants are more likely to receive greater monetary compensation if they persist longer.

5.2.4 Economic Cost Concerns

On the distributive aspect, economic costs are also another important factor shaping the compensation outcome. A prevalent view for explaining the application of buying stability is that the government usually apply monetary incentives instrumentally as a concession to deter the potential activists (Benney, 2016; Lee & Zhang, 2013). However, not all monetary claims are satisfied due to the cost-efficient reasons. In specific, in facing large-scale compensation claims, government often might be more sensitive and cautious under the economic cost pressure. For instance, when workers pursue demands for compensation such as overtime stipulated by the law, the large-scale monetary compensation claims could lead to the relocation or even bankruptcy of some enterprises, which is less desired by local officials as they want to favor the interests of employers to protect local economic development. This strategy is also reflected in the September 11 Victims Compensation Funds established by the government to prevent the enterprise bankrupt by protecting them from victims' large compensation lawsuits (Hadfield, 2008).

In dealing with medical disputes, similar logic persists. Solving medical disputes requires human resource input from both mediators and hospital representatives. On the one hand, small compensation claims are associated with less economic cost and less resource demand. Therefore, satisfying small-scale compensation claims could reduce mediators' time allocation and resources and contribute to a high mediation rate, which is also desirable for the organizational interests of the hospitals. On the other hand, hospitals are more likely to give priority to solving large compensation claims such as equipping with more professional resources including legal consultants and staff, which makes the bargaining process more difficult. For instance, Chen and Zhang's study (2019) finds that medical disputes that involve large compensation claims are more likely to elicit the local government's intervention in collective deliberation and joint efforts from various government authorities. Hence, different coping strategies under the logic of the "divide and conquer" are applied for addressing small- and large-scale compensation requests. I hypothesize that in contrast to small compensation claims, large compensation requests are less likely to be satisfied.

To summarize, by examining the factors shaping compensation distribution, this chapter developed a conceptual framework for understanding the strategies of compensation distribution based on three recoupling logics. The first logic emphasizes the importance of pursuing the public perception of distributive justice that combines social appropriateness and rules to enhance organizational legitimacy. The second logic emphasizes discretionary power in judging cases by applying informal rules to identify potential troublemakers to maintain social stability. The third logic explains that monetary compensation is also constrained by economic cost concerns. Mediators need to balance various principles simultaneously; therefore, the interaction among various principles could be important to understanding the compensation distribution.

5.2.5 Where Does the Money Come from?

Before we examine the rationale of compensation, it is necessary to explain who pays in the end for the medical disputes. Since China has a strong public hospital system, medical dispute compensation is also unique through both formal and informal channels.

Instituted to ease the compensation pressure placed upon the hospitals, medical liability insurance was recently convened as a mechanism for shifting responsibility by allowing an insurance company to pay compensation in medical disputes and to avoid direct contact between the patients and hospitals. Medical liability insurance is a new and immature industry in China, in contrast to many developed countries. The invention of medical liability insurance is a side product of all-compassing social stability maintenance mechanism in response to the rising medical disputes. As Zhang Zhi'an, the vice president of the Jiangtai insurance Broker Company, commented,

> Under the logic of stability maintenance, medical disputes are no longer the disputes between hospitals and patients, but patients and government … Since the introduction of medical liability insurance, it has shouldered the social management function. It is not merely ordinary commercial insurance, which simply relies on compensation mechanisms and rate leverage. It was packed up with the function of social management as perform as a quasi-public good.[4]

[4] See, for instance, Medical liability insurance helps build an integrated medical risk sharing mechanism, http://xw.cbimc.cn/2015-05/13/content_154749.htm, accessed on October 2, 2023.

Since 2002, the C city has become the pioneer in encouraging hospitals, regardless of ownership, to be covered by insurance. Based on this directive, most hospitals (mainly public hospitals) are covered by medical liability insurance schemes. By the end of 2019, tertiary hospitals (all public hospitals) in the fieldwork city are all covered by medical liability insurance, and the coverage rate in secondary hospitals is also as high as 90%. Likewise, in Ningxia province (Western China), from 2012 to 2015, the above-mentioned Jiangtai Insurance Broker company provided compensation of up to 35 million RMB to 680 medical dispute cases with an average processing time of five working days. For instance, in one dispute that involved hospital violence by publicly displaying the coffin in the lobby of the hospital, the insurance company facilitated the mediation committee in finalizing the amount of compensation and provided the compensation on the same day afternoon without delay.[5] The efficient compensation suppliance has facilitated the dispute resolution in a timely manner.

However, the drawbacks of medical liability insurance are also obvious. First, the imbalanced insurance coverage between public and private hospitals is apparent. The coverage rate among private hospitals is low, and the latter de facto have a lower capability to pay compensation. The insurance companies are wary of the frequent occurrence of medical disputes involving private hospitals, and therefore only a small group of insurance companies are willing to provide insurance services to these private hospitals, resulting in a small coverage rate and high pricing. Second, the medical liability insurance premiums were up to a fixed ceiling of coverage. For instance, one tertiary hospital (referred to as F) spent 1.2 million RMB annually on insurance. Yet, it is much less than the monetary compensation they have fulfilled per year. When the current premium fails to cover the compensation for the current year, it would pass the cost on to the hospitals in the following calendar year. During the fieldwork, the interviewee commented it could not address their needs by counting on the insurance only. Hospitals would also rely on other channels to fill the resource gap.

Hence, given the frequent occurrence of medical disputes as well as disruptive actions in the hospitals, each hospital also has innovated its way of using monetary ways to address medical disputes. In most cases, the compensation issue could be settled internally by hospitals and doctors collectively. As a penalty, the involved department and doctor would be denied awarding honorable rewards and bonuses in the same year. For cases that involve large compensation, higher health authorities and local government would intervene (Chen & Zhang, 2019). As such, hospitals, health authorities, as well as local governments are also under the financial burden to provide compensation for the disputants.

---

[5] Ibid.

5.2.6 Data and Variables

This chapter draws on both qualitative and quantitative methods to observe the rationale in compensation distribution practices in China. I collected medical dispute cases processed between 2013 and 2017 from one location in the fieldwork city. In total, 762 case files were documented for data processing; 665 cases remained after excluding 80 cases that did not achieve agreement between hospitals and patients; and 17 cases were transferred again to the litigation channel.

I focus on examining the principles of compensation distribution, theorizing the rationale for compensation distribution by considering the perception of justice, political, and economic cost concerns. The key dependent variable was measured by the finalized amount of monetary compensation received by the patients. I also use the binary dependent variable of "claim satisfaction" to compare the claim requested by the patients and the final compensation received. If the monetary compensation claims accounts for 80% of the finalized compensation (20% as a buffer monetary compensation),[6] the claim would be categorized as "satisfied." For instance, if a patient requested 1,000 RMB for compensation, the claim would be categorized as satisfied (claim satisfaction = 1) if the final compensation was greater than 800 RMB.[7] I did not use the previous dependent variables because small-scale compensateon claims are naturally associated with a lower compensation amount.

The independent variable includes the severity of the medical facts it was positively associated with the public perception of justice and leads to higher compensation. The case-level data contain the following three types of medical results: death, disability, and absent medical results. Increased levels of medical severity increase the possibility of receiving compensation. The data also includes whether the case has gone through an external medical examination. If patients agree to seek expert reviews, more systematic and subjective judgements could be provided with written reports by professional groups. Since the People's Mediation Committee reflected distributive justice in semi-legal institutions, the severity of the medical results might be associated with the amount of compensation received.

Meanwhile, discretion may also apply to compensation redistribution due to political concerns associated with showing concession to troublemakers. The persistence of the individual was an important indicator of seeking positive responses from officials. This captures the resources that individuals would spend in the bargaining process. Therefore, this chapter uses the *bargain time* (unit: days) as a proxy for the persistence of patients. The bargain time is calculated as the overall time spent in each case and quantifies the time effort spent by hospitals and patients in managing a single case under the facilitation of the mediation committee (three-party negotiation and bargaining process). The bargain time reveals the level of perseverance of a patient in addressing a medical dispute. The more perseverance a patient has,

---

[6] Various thresholds (20%, 30%, 35%, and 40%) are also tested. This study draws the 20% threshold from the interviews. Patients could expect their compensation claims to be partially fulfilled, usually ranging from 10 to 30%.

[7] Threshold of 90% is also applied to test the results.

the more time he/she spends in the mediating process to achieve a desired outcome, which would receive more compensation, ceteris paribus.

Next, economic cost concerns also shape various compensation distribution outcomes. The independent variable representing economic concerns is a binary variable of the scale of the compensation. The centralized bargaining channel may be more cautious in addressing large-scale compensation than addressing small-scale claims. Due to the institutional design, the mediation committee introduces the institutional design of dividing compensation claims into the following two groups: more or less than 30,000 RMB. If the compensation claims are less than 30,000 RMB, the procedure of compensation distribution could be settled privately between patients and hospitals without further examination. Small-scale compensation claims, which are associated with less institutional screening and attention, are more likely to be satisfied to increase the cost-efficiency of the mediation channels.

I also include a set of other variables at both hospital and individual level. This study controls for both hospital- and individual-level attributes that may contribute to the final compensation distribution. Regarding the hospital-level attributes, scholars have argued that there are nested interests between the government and organizations due to economic concerns (Lee & Zhang, 2013). The rank of hospitals is China also indicates their resources and administrative ranking. Public hospitals (up to 90% of mediation cases), which are funded and operated by the government, shared vested interests and natural bonds with the local government (Eggleston et al., 2010). Based on the three-tier health delivery service in China (Chen, 2009), the ranking of hospitals is coded as tertiary hospitals (3), secondary hospitals (2), and community health centers (1) under the hospital-level variable. On the individual-level data, I also include the control variables include the fixed-year effect and individual characteristics of the disputant, including gender, age, province and *hukou* (户口). The *hukou* information describes whether the claimant is a local resident (Fig. 5.1). Compared to local residents, non-local disputants are often considered underprivileged social groups with limited resources (e.g. see Michelson, 2007), which might affect their bargaining power in the mediation process. The age factor is also controlled in medical dispute resolution as younger patients (e.g., in their 30s) are more likely to receive more compensation as it also takes compensation for their dependents into considerations. Table 5.1 reports the full list of variables applied in the study and their summary statistics.

5.3 Findings

"In most cases, money matters."[8]

---

[8] Interview with a senior mediator in September 2017.

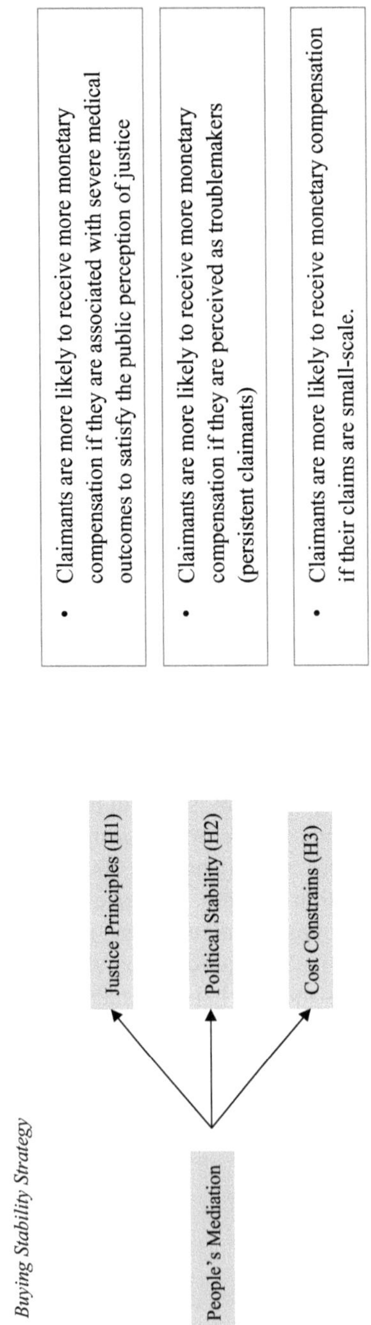

Fig. 5.1 Conceptual Framework of rationale for compensation distribution

Table 5.1 Variable Summary Statistics

	Observations	Mean	Std. Dev	Min	Max
Compensation (log) (RMB)	665	9.08	2.78	0	14.4
Claim satisfied	665	0.20	0.40	0	1
Medical result	665	2.56	0.81	1	3
Bargain time (days)	665	15.35	26.46	1	323
Gender	665	0.50	0.50	0	1
Age (years)	665	43.79	23.91	0	94
External consultation	665	1.21	0.41	1	2
Hospital level	665	2.07	0.87	0	3
Local resident	665	0.61	0.49	0	1
Province	665	15.28	6.80	1	24

5.3.1 Empirical Results

The analysis covers 665 mediated medical dispute cases. The results of the statistical models are presented in Table 5.2. Models 1 and 2 examine the regression of the amount of compensation (in its natural log form) associated with medical results over five years. Model 2 contains the hospital-level control variables, including the hospital level and whether an external expert review was performed. Models 3 and 4 regress the compensation and bargain time to examine the government-led mediation response toward troublemakers. Model 5 includes all independent and control variables. The results regarding the quantities of interest remained statistically significant across the various models, showing a positive and significant relationship between severe medical outcomes (e.g., death and disability) and the receipt of a higher monetary compensation. This relationship partially explains the rationale embedded in the decision-making logic based on distributive justice in determining the compensation amount. Consistent with a previous study, the mediation channel acts as a semi-legal institution aiming to maintain social justice based on the general perception of justice. The severity of the medical results is an important factor in determining the final compensation outcomes. In Fig. 5.3 I use a simulation of the medical results by including the hospital-level characteristics and personal attributes, such as local residence, at their observed values and setting the coefficients based on the linear regression in the full model (Model 5). The simulation results show that compensation is negatively associated with medical disputes when the degree of the medical severity decreases, which cannot be attributed to other factors, including demographic, medical and hospital variables.

The persistence of the patient is also positively associated with receiving a greater monetary compensation. The findings remain statistically significant across all models. One unit (day) accumulated in a day spent prior to the mediation channel led to a 0.1% (**) increase in the final compensation. The longer the history of the

Table 5.2 Regression analysis results regarding monetary compensation

	Model 1	Model 2	Model 3	Model 4	Model 5
Medical-outcome (death)	2.708***	2.380***			2.402***
	(0.242)	(0.254)			(0.254)
Medical-outcome (disability)	3.780***	3.635***			3.625***
	(0.323)	(0.323)			(0.319)
Bargain time (3 Parties)			0.019***	0.009**	0.010**
			(0.004)	(0.003)	(0.003)
Gender	−0.428**	−0.405**	0.063	0.017	−0.404**
	(0.201)	(0.198)	(0.213)	(0.207)	(0.197)
Age	−0.005	−0.005	−0.001	−0.002	−0.005
	(0.004)	(0.004)	(0.005)	(0.005)	(0.004)
Local resident	−0.211	−0.19	−0.409*	−0.354	−0.178
	(0.225)	(0.225)	(0.243)	(0.238)	(0.224)
Expert review		0.789***		1.476***	0.525*
		(0.264)		(0.278)	(0.270)
Hospital level		0.05		0.121	0.019
		(0.115)		(0.119)	(0.117)
Year of medical disputes	Yes	Yes	Yes	Yes	Yes
Constant	8.718***	8.749***	11.981***	11.993***	8.580***
	(0.436)	(0.480)	(0.301)	(0.401)	(0.482)
Observations	665	665	665	665	665
R2	0.216	0.227	0.065	0.105	0.234
Adjusted R2	0.204	0.213	0.052	0.09	0.219
Residual Std. Error	2.479 (df = 654)	2.465 (df = 652)	2.704 (df = 655)	2.650 (df = 654)	2.456 (df = 651)
F Statistic	17.972*** (df = 10; 654)	15.962*** (df = 12; 652)	5.067*** (df = 9; 655)	6.972*** (df = 11; 653)	15.286*** (df = 13; 651)

*p < 0.1; **p < 0.05; ***p < 0.01

medical disputes also signals the patient's persistence in realizing his/her compensation claim. In the mediation channel, there is pressure to efficiently settle cases with long conflict histories. The coefficient is positive and significant at the 0.05 level, which is consistent with the hypothesis and the findings of previous studies. To measure the expected value of our quantities of interest (time and medical severity), a similar approach was applied to observe the expected value of compensation for various levels of medical severity. Figure 5.2 plots the expected value of compensation (log) for different time durations. This analysis tests the changing expected value of compensation with each increase in the bargain time from 0 to 180 days (half of a year), while the other variables maintained their observed values. The figure demonstrates the positive effect of the bargain time on the receipt of a higher monetary compensation.

These findings confirm Hypotheses 1 and 2. Regarding the justice principles, the analysis demonstrates that negative medical outcomes (disability and death) are more likely to lead to higher amounts of compensation to satisfy the public perception of distributive justice. This finding is consistent with the hypothesis that the People's

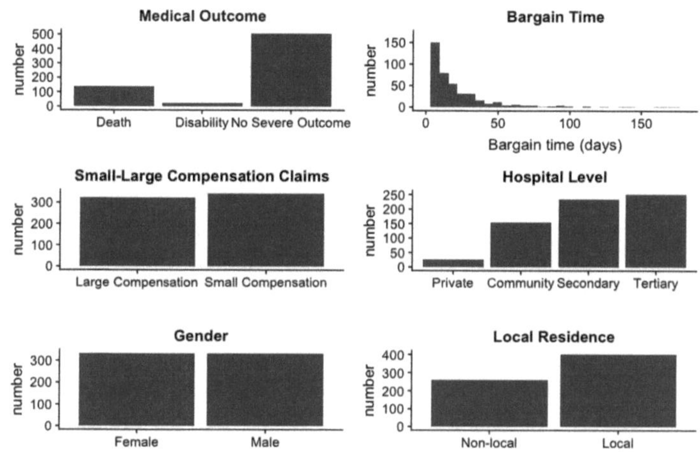

Fig. 5.2 The distribution of key variables

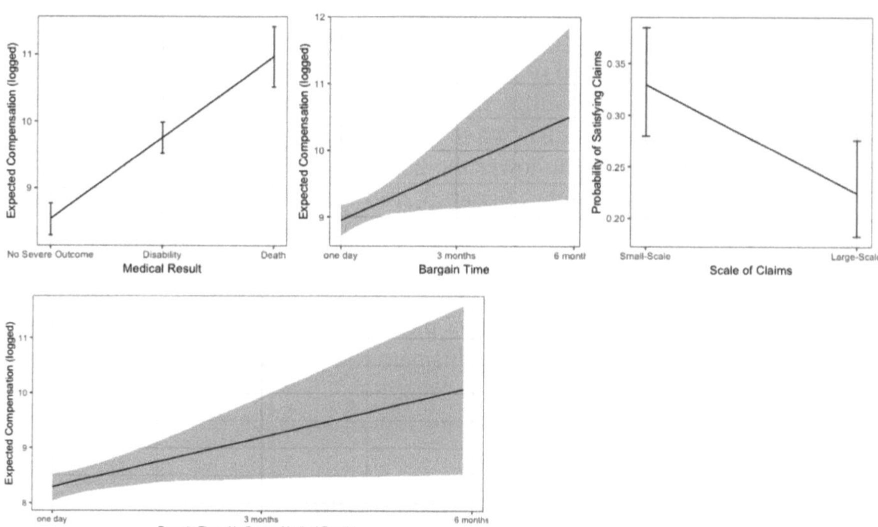

Fig. 5.3 Expected value of compensation, medical results and expected value of compensation and duration (95% confidence intervals)

Mediation plays a crucial role in making decisions based on both formal and informal rules. Meanwhile, regarding the political stability concern factors, troublemakers or specifically persistent claimants who spend a longer time bargaining with the hospital counterpart are more likely to receive a higher compensation. Compensation is more likely to be distributed to show concessions toward troublemakers for stability maintenance purposes. Additionally, it is possible that there could be correlation between the medical results and bargain time. For example, a long bargain time may be due to a complicated injury or procrastination. Therefore, this study used cases that are not associated with medical injuries to test the results. The results remain robust (see Fig. 5.3).

Notably, regarding the control variables, the expert review remains consistently statistically significant. However, only a few cases sought expert consultations to confirm medical malpractice (26%). It is common in China for compensation to be distributed without identifying the facts related to the medical case. The reasons for this trend are complicated. Learning the facts of a medical dispute through an expert review could be risky for the patient, who could lose the advantage in the bargaining process through confirmation that there was no medical malpractice. Only a few patients would resort to an expert review. Regarding the personal-level attributes, gender (female) is more likely associated with a higher compensation, indicating that inconsistent compensation is distributed across cases.

Subsequently, this chapter focuses on a logit regression of small- or large-scale compensation claims (Table 5.3). Models 6 and 7 regress the claim satisfaction on the scale of the claims and bargain time, and model 7 includes the personal attributes of gender, local resident variables and the fixed-year effect. Model 8 includes the hospital-level control variables. Model 9 includes all independent and control variables.

The small-scale compensation claims show positive and consistent significant correlations with the likelihood of claim satisfaction, and this result remains robust in all models. This finding confirms the hypothesis that small-scale compensation claims are more likely to be satisfied due to cost constraints or economic concerns. This analysis also finds that the lower the hospital level, the higher the likelihood of satisfying the patients' claims. Figure 5.2 also shows the effect of small-scale compensation on the possibility of claims being satisfied.

Overall speaking, inconsistent patterns are found in the compensation distribution such that small-scale claims and troublemakers receive greater responsiveness. Limited information is known regarding the hidden mechanism of the mediation process. Qualitative evidence may help elucidate how various principles are weighted in the buying stability strategy.

5.3.2 Qualitative Evidence: Buying Stability for ALL?

The fieldwork shows that in contrast to courts, through the mediation channel, mediators could incorporate various considerations into their compensation distribution,

Table 5.3 Logit regression analysis results regarding claim satisfaction

	Model 6	Model 7	Model 8	Model 9
Below 30 k	0.608***	0.607***	0.499**	0.540***
	(0.177)	(0.180)	(0.196)	(0.198)
Bargain time (3 Parties)	0.001**			0.001*
	(0.000)			(0.000)
Gender		−0.238	−0.197	−0.200
		(0.178)	(0.182)	(0.183)
Age		−0.002	−0.003	−0.003
		(0.004)	(0.004)	(0.004)
Local resident		0.114	0.160	0.129
		(0.196	(0.199)	(0.200)
Hospital Level			−0.225**	−0.233**
			(0.109)	(0.110)
Expert review			−0.134	−0.100
			(0.262)	(0.262)
Year of Medical Disputes	No	Yes	Yes	Yes
Constant	−1.362***	−13.573	−13.073	−13.163
	(0.14)	(1.04)	(1.063)	(1.06)
Observations	665	665	665	665
Log likelihood	–388.392	–381.527	–379.070	–377.230
Akaike Inf. Crit	782.783	783.053	782.139	780.468

*p < 0.1; **p < 0.05; ***p < 0.01

including reflecting the public perception of justice, responding to the claims of persistent disputants, as well as increasing organizational efficacy. Compared to judges, the mediators' role in dispute resolution is much more active and enjoys more discretional power. There are often three reasons that explain the behaviors of the mediators. First, compensation distribution becomes a crucial and core element in dispute resolution, and the disputants' perception of justice and satisfaction towards the medical institutions largely depends on the redistributive results in the compensation distribution process. The mediators prefer to promote distributive justice to satisfy the masses. Without a sufficient understanding of the law and regulations, many disputants have unrealistic expectations towards the mediation channel and mediators and misunderstand the medical dispute resolution process.

For instance, one 76-year-old patient with cancer died on the operating table. The patient's family asked for a total of 600,000 RMB compensation, while the hospital denied the request and only agreed to offer symbolic compensation for humanitarian reasons.[9] The patient's family was agitated and accused the hospital

[9] Based on author's fieldnote.

of lacking informed consent for disclosing the risks before and during the surgery. The case went through the external expert review and reached the conclusion that the involved doctor did not emphasize the risk of the surgery and the case could be compensated referring to the first level of medical malpractice by providing a one-time 300,000 RMB compensation (half of the original claim). Although the operation was based on the doctor's best judgement and the patient's family signed the informed consent notice, it failed to highlight the risks that it may become a factor causing the patient's injuries or death. The mediation committee spent great efforts to persuade the hospital to provide compensation for cases that involved the death of patients. At last, the involved hospital agreed to provide one-time settlement compensation and the patient families highly praised the mediation channels for their hard work in protecting their rights.

One mediator explained,

> The patient or their family members often held the belief that someone must have to be responsible for this tragedy. Otherwise, they would find the system unfair or fail to protect their interests or assumes that the hospitals were covering up. It is their perception of justice.[10]

It illustrates the difference between the law and the traditional notion of justice which lays the foundation of the mediation. As He's study (2021) shows, in China, the litigants' attitudes towards civil justice are under the influence of "distributive justice". That is, whether the outcome favored to their sides plays a decisive role in their perception and assessments of the court system (He & Feng, 2021, Gallagher & Wang, 2011). The outcome-oriented disputants are more concerned with their personal efficacy in the legal system, instead of procedural justice. To some extent, mediation channels converge the procedural justice as well as the public perception of distributed justice by emphasizing the outcomes. By distributing monetary compensation towards the disputants, the mediation channel aimed to increase the disputants' personal efficacy in the mediation channel by responding to their grievances. For the mediators, in addition to following written rules, informal norms sometimes were a crucial criterion in shaping the compensation distribution process and often justified the utilization of discretion. Through the process, almost all disputants could receive compensation, though varied in amount. By doing so, mediators focused on distributive justice to satisfy the public perception or imagination of justice. As a result, for many disputants, mediation is "fairer" than the courts as it is outcome-oriented and partially reflects the public perception of distributive justice.

It is also notable that there are a few cases in which disputants walk out without taking any form of compensation as they are completely convinced by the mediator, which also demonstrated the efficacy of the mediation channels to address the tie through persuasion and legal literacy. For instance, the mediator also proudly told the author that many disputes are caused by misunderstanding and distrust between patients and doctors. They (as mediators) helped to explain the uncertainties in medicine and relieved the pain of the loss of their beloved. Some patient's families decided not to sue the doctor.

---

[10] Interview with the mediator in August 2017.

Table 5.4 Background of the Mediators

Categories		N
Contract type	Full time	100
	Part time	23
Age	Avg. age	54
Job background	Medical service	56
	Law enforcement	19
	Other	25

Second, the mediation process may still inevitably involve the exercise of discretionary power. Social stability concern also prompt mediators to allocate more time and efforts to target population and difficult cases. While addressing compensation claims, mediators usually categorize the scale of compensation to identify the potential threat involved and cost incurred. Based on this direction, according to the mediators, four scenarios may trigger the discretionary power associated with greater attention from the mediation committee: (1) cases involving large-scale compensation, (2) cases involving children or pitiable patients, (3) cases with severe medical outcomes, and (4) cases involving multiple patients, which may lead to collective actions.

Mediators' political background and good government connections help them to identify sensitive cases in a preventive manner. Table 5.4 presents the career backgrounds of 100 full-time mediators in the fieldwork city. We find that 75 of them were employed in or worked for party organs, including public hospitals, police bureaus, and legal bureaus. Their political backgrounds and working backgrounds ensured that they were a respected and credible workforce. For example, nineteen former policemen had become mediators after retirement. They used to be street-level bureaucratic workers from the law enforcement department, which made them good at restoring social order and refraining patients from applying disruptive actions. These politically minded mediators must balance various interests among hospitals and patients and satisfy the social stability maintenance goal of the government. Mediators often prioritize sensitive and difficult cases and manage them cautiously by applying concession or discretion. For instance, a child patient involved in a medical dispute may attract the attention and moral indignation of the family, society, and the media.[11] It should be attached with great importance.

Likewise, nonlocal disputants are often carefully treated carefully. For instance, Mr. W, who is a non-local resident who suspected the failure in his surgery said.

> It took me half a day to come to the C city to settle the medical dispute. I do not how many times I need to commute between C and J (hometown) to get this done. It costs me a lot time and efforts. At first, I suspect that the mediators would cover up and aside with the hospitals considering I am not a local resident. But the mediators treat me with kind and make me feel less inferior to the hospitals.[12]

[11] Interview with the director of a mediation committee in August 2016.

[12] Based on author's fieldnote in the Mediation committee in September 2017.

From the mediators' perspective, non-local residents who seek health services in C city often have a higher expectation of the medical results, hence it often would lead to dissatisfaction. It would lead them to blame the doctors, the hospitals, then the system at large. Hence, we need to treat them with specific care to increase and apply discretional power when possible. The proactive role of the mediation works as leverage allowing for a balancing of power relations between the hospital and patients.

Meanwhile, petty money is occasionally distributed due to the efficacy and social stability reasons. If a patient is persistent in pursuing a medical dispute, pressure may be felt by the mediators and hospitals during the bargaining process, forcing them to accept a better deal in terms of compensation. For example, a typical case occurred in 2016 and lasted for one year, creating headache for hospitals.

Feeling the inefficiency of the medical treatment provided, one woman frequently "harassed" one secondary-level hospital and her doctor for more than a year. She visited the hospital every day and sit in the doctor's office while without violent behaviors. Yet her presence has made the doctor feel uncomfortable and disrupted the order in the hospitals. The doctor called the police many times, but the only thing police could do is to send her home as there is no severe disruptive actions. The next day, the woman showed up at the doctor's office on time at 8 o'clock again. Her "nonviolent" behaviors pushed the hospital to call for mediation committee to respond. Through mediation, the mediator convinced the woman to stop her behaviors through long-term persuasion as well as distributing material benefits. In exchange, the hospital finally compensated her 10,000 RMB to "buy peace". The mediator commented, "You can just tell from the document that it is none of the business or responsibility of the doctors and hospitals. We paid anyway; you know; she was just crazy.[13]"

The mediators may consider persistent patients as "troublemakers" as they will not give up until paid and less likely to be punished by existing regulations. A case may not be a medical malpractice case from a professional's perspective, but compensation is still distributed due to non-medical factors, such as culture, to show sympathy for others and address stability concerns. It may not only be due to the fear of escalation into severe confrontations but also because of organizational interest in saving the resources and efforts of both hospitals and mediators. These stability concerns are closely associated with the outcomes of medical disputes and sometimes outweigh professional judgements and medical facts.

Third, mediators have confined their discretional power in compensation distributing to the minimum, only towards small-scale claims associated with low economic costs and low political threats from the mediators' perspective. Different from the original notion of "buying stability", the mediators have clearer standings and preferences in limiting the application of buying stability to avoid increasing the personal efficacy in influencing the outcomes. People's Mediation institution pays more attention towards institutionalizing the compensation distribution to make it consistent across cases. For instance, from January to May 2015, a medical dispute

[13] Interview with a mediator in October 2017.

for a cardiac surgery for a child failed to achieve mediation between the patient and hospital. The patient's family requested 482, 600 RMB in compensation, but no agreement has been reached, which clearly failed to be explained under the framework of buying stability. The mediator stated the following:

> For such large compensation claims, if we compensate for no reason, it will not only damage the interests of the hospitals but also set a bad role model for the rest. And the patients would also be concerned that maybe the hospital hides something they don't know. Therefore, we also encourage the patients to go through the lawsuits. We pay no heed to trifles but are serious with big things (小事糊涂，大事不可以糊涂).

Government officials, under cadre promotion pressure, are more likely to apply inconsistent compensation or usually over-compensation occurs to satisfy the patient's demands (Chen & Zhang, 2019). In comparison, as the mediation channel has developed a high degree of formality and professionalism, compensating for no reason could harm their legitimacy and organizational interests. The organizational aim of the mediation committee is to institutionalize the dispute resolution process and prompt consistent compensation distribution. If mediation fails to carry out consistent compensation claims, their status and qualifications will be questioned. Therefore, mediators first screen for potential threats not based on troublemaking tactics but on the cost of the disputes. If it is a large compensation case, more efforts and attention are attributed to protecting the organizational interests. In small compensation cases, discretion is more likely to be applied in exchange for improving the efficiency of the case processing.

During the mediation process, in addition to negotiating with the patients, mediators may also face subtle pressure from hospitals, which may limit their discretionary power in compensating patients. As shown in the figure, this analysis also found that the lower the hospital level, the higher the likelihood that patients' claims will be satisfied (Table 5.2). Mediators face strong institutional pressure from the hospitals. The interviewees (patients) indicated a changing atmosphere among hospitals and their attitudes toward medical disputes. Some leading high-level public hospitals are becoming more sophisticated and cautious about addressing medical disputes by equipping themselves with better monitoring equipment (CCTV), security teams, insurance representatives, lawyers, and social work professionals. Monitoring equipment helps to prevent the occurrence of hospital violence and reduce crimes, thereby maintaining hospital security. Besides the "hardware" innovation, hospitals are more willing to support doctors and are unwilling to compensate patients for unidentified medical cases in large-scale compensation cases, as doing so may affect their reputation.

For instance, mediators said that they were often shocked by facing so many lawyers in mediation conferences. Getting hospitals to provide large compensation is becoming increasingly difficult. They provide documents indicating there is no precedent of compensation distribution, and often state that they cannot make an exception. This has often tied mediators' hands and prevented the achievement of agreement between the disputing parties. Strong institutional power lies in the hands of public hospital to influence the compensation outcome.

In comparison, when private hospitals were involved, they were often shorthanded when it came to the bargaining process. According to a mediator, private hospitals are far more likely to accept deals proposed by mediators. Private hospitals have limited resources to address medical disputes, and most are neither entitled to nor willing to buy medical liability insurance. They usually do not have full-time lawyers, nor administrative or full-time staff working on dispute resolution. It is far easier for mediators to persuade them and to arrive at an agreement. From the private hospitals' perspective, the People's Mediation Committee often represented the government, rendering high authority and power. Thus, private hospitals often take a humble approach. They are far more likely to comply with the mediators' pressure to accept the compensation outcome. In occasional cases, the mediators "pressured" hospital representatives to accept the compensation outcome through utilizing their deep connections with the health supervisory agency. For private hospitals, maintaining sound relations with the government and its partners is an important goal. Otherwise, they cannot afford repetitive meetings, negotiations, or routinized spot checks led by supervising bodies.

The role of the private sector, especially the insurance sector, may warrant some attention in explaining the compensation distribution outcome embedded in the mediation process as well. Since the insurance sector is afraid of exceeding premium limits, they also perform a supervisory role in decreasing cases of overcompensation, driven by monetary incentives and job responsibility. They usually participate in the mediation process in two ways. First, some insurance companies dispatch insurance representatives stationed in the hospitals to deal with the patients directly. They would assist the hospitals in absorbing and processing patients' demands, preparing documents pertaining to medical disputes, and granting compensation. Second, the insurance sector also selectively participates in the mediation process. According to the committee chief,

> For compensation exceeding 100,000 RMB, cases that might cause mass incidents, complicated cases that may attract popular attention, they (insurance representative) would participate in the case study conference and expert consulting meeting. Sometimes, they would also join in the communication process with the patients.[14]

By delegating the compensation distribution responsibility to People's Mediation, the organizational interests of the mediation committee are intertwined with government priorities. First, mediators aim to make consistent compensation decisions and, therefore, refrain from over-responding to claimants' requests. This approach reduces the social stability maintenance cost by refraining from the application of the buying stability strategy. Meanwhile, mediators aim to combine procedural justice and distributive justice in the dispute resolution process. Mediators not only take the responsibility attribution into consideration but also take the "medical severity" or the pain of the patients into account. By doing so, it also increased the personnel efficacy in dispute resolution, which would enhance their satisfaction towards the mediation channel and the associated result.

[14] Interview with the Chief of Mediation Committee in August 2017 and follow up interview in June 2020.

Additionally, delegating to People's Mediation provides the disputants an alternative dispute resolution channel. This channel prevents the government from its direct involvement in social disputes and avoids blame. It is also physically "separate" the patients and hospitals to avoid the escalation of disputes and prevent the occurrence of disruptive actions. This channel performs as an information collective channel to identify potential threats and grievances, which calls for joint intervention from all relevant departments. For instance, once during the mediation process, the father of the deceased daughter yelled and slapped the table from time to time. He took a heart emergency medicine in front of the hospital representative to show his vulnerability and poor health, and threatened to meet the dean of the hospital with a knife. According to the 25th article of the People's Mediation law, any disputes that may cause criminal or create disturbances need to be reported to the local public security office.[15] The mediators soon contacted the local police. The father only came back to sanity and was back at the negotiation table after the local police officer's persuasion.

The chief of one mediation committee commented, "We have strong support from other government organizations, such as the police, health bureau, and neighborhood community. Once they (patients) threaten to go to extremes, we would step in."[16] Through the integrated stability maintenance system, the mediators could prevent the occurrence of collective actions by closely monitoring the progress of the disputes and collaborate with other coercive forces as well as social workers to intervene.

Taken together, both quantitative and qualitative evidence consistently suggest the political, social, and economic rationale in compensation distribution and how the introduction of the mediation committee applied an updated buying stability mechanism to promote the public perception of justice in dispute resolution. To exercise buying stability 2.0, the mediators usually categorize the scale of the compensation to identify the potential threat and cost embedded. Their political background and good connection with the government help them identify sensitive cases. Meanwhile, mediators apply various tackling strategies. Small-scale compensation claims could be addressed using a discretion or leniency approach to enhance efficiency and show sympathy towards the patients to reflect morality and confirm the personal efficacy in the dispute resolution systems. Large-scale compensation claims could require more resources and time allocation to the cases. The latter could pay special attention to applying the rule of justice to avoid potential troubles by making consistent and legally binding decisions. Mediators are also sophisticated and can adopt a two-step processing method to identify problematic cases. This approach protects the organizational interests of hospitals and mediation committees. It contrasts the belief of "big disruption, big resolution" (大闹大解决) in resorting to buying stability as suggested by earlier scholars. This chapter finds that compensation distribution is very cautious and institutionalized to promote a consistent distribution pattern, which helps decrease the stability maintenance cost, satisfies political stability concerns, and adheres to the distributive justice concept.

---

15 See, for instance, People's Mediation Law of the People's Republic of China, https://www.gov.cn/flfg/2010-08/29/content_1691209.htm, accessed on October 20, 2023.

16 Interview with a mediator in July 2017.

5.4 The Limits of Bargained Authoritarianism

Facing the mounting social disputes, the government increasingly applied monetary compensation as a solution to readdress citizens' grievances and maintain social order. Buying stability is an effective non-coercive strategy the government applied to deal with the rightful resistance. However, too much reliance on buying stability may endanger the legitimacy of the rulers generate high economic costs, and even encourage the interest-seeking behaviors of the troublemakers. Hence, in recent years, semi-formal institutions at the local government level have been increasingly revitalized to address all types of social disputes as well as compensation distribution problems. The political space to apply disruptive tactics to bargain with the government is slimmed under the political tightened control. This approach further signals that the regime has developed all-encompassing social stability maintenance schemes by including all necessary political authorities and even semi-formal institutions to prevent and contain potential threats.

To avoid being directly involved in dispute resolution as well as to promote consistent outcomes, the government delegated the role to the mediation institutions. Mediation institutions not only regulate social relations between public institutions and citizens but also become the venue of central bargaining channels, acting as a preventive strategy to use carrots in exchange for social stability. The mediation institution institutionalizes the compensation distribution process while remaining flexible in resorting to discretion as a way of co-opting tools in cases that might lead to mass incidents or popular attention.

The chapter proposes a framework to uncover the rationale of compensation distribution, which broadens the understanding of applying buying stability in China. The study suggests that the outcomes of buying stability are shaped by the perception of distributive justice, political stability concerns, and economic cost considerations. The institution of People's Mediation could successfully balance various conflicting goals through the intermediary role of the mediators. The mediators, as the gatekeepers, were more responsive towards small-scale compensation claims, cases associated with severe medical results, and persistent claimants. Meanwhile, the mediators also refrain from the use of buying stability to avoid providing incentives for troublemakers to apply disruptive actions. They often perceive large-scale claims as potential threats to their organizational interests and reputation and are afraid that over-compensation may lead to the diffusion of disruptive tactics. Taken together, it contributed to the institutionalization of buying stability to reduce the economic burden of the local government, as well as maintain the social order.

However, the bargained authoritarianism is not flawless, and the limitations of buying stability are three-folded. First, the quasi-officials as mediators become the gatekeepers at the local government to balance various conflicting goals. In the short term, it helps the local government achieve its social government goals. Yet, the sustainability and efficacy of the mediation committee are contingent upon the incentives and qualifications of semi-officials, which is difficult to control and monitor. For instance, existing mediators are usually in their late 50s, who are loyal to the political system and have established strong social ties among the community. In comparison, the young generation of the mediation are often professionally trained as the social workers, who detached from the community and lacked the authority among the residents, which would make the mediation and compensation bargaining process more difficult. As some full-time mediators are still on the payroll of the government, it would also make the expenditure in social stability maintenance under heavy burden, and less likely to sustain in a longer time frame.

Second, it also reflects the public perception of justice among ordinary citizens and the half-halted of the rule of law in China. In recent decades, legal institutions, such as courts, have been highly occupied and overwhelmed by social disputes, reflecting the dilemma faced by juridical workers. The regime thus relied increasingly heavily on semi-legal mediation institutions to run more smoothly and efficiently by redirecting discontented citizens to the mediation committee to settle for compensation. It is likely that this trend will continue by emphasizing the application of discretion, traditional norms, and informal rules, which further downplay the roles of the courts and the judiciary system, as well as the professional organizations. The institution of People's Mediation is like a Band-Aid in contemporary China to absorb all of the grievances and discontent, allowing political institutions to apply a more pragmatic approach to managing social disputes. However, it dampens the basic spirit of the rule of law and increases the government's burden in dispute resolution.

Drawing on the prior studies, this study revisits the scholarly accounts and suggests that the citizens took a pragmatic attitude by resorting to rule- and law-consciousness flexibly and orienting on the distributive outcomes they received. The citizens, though widely applying the narratives of right and legal rules, their perception of justice and the rule of law is still contingent upon their efficacy, morality, and outcomes they received in the system. Through the fieldwork, I often find that the public perception of justice is largely shaped by the outcomes, morality, and efficacy of their role in receiving material interests in the dispute resolution process. Citizens adopt flexible and pragmatic attitudes towards the perception of justice by emphasizing the outcomes they received in the process of interacting with the state as well as their agents. The public has a limited understanding of the law, and largely decides "right and wrong" by drawing on the traditional notions of morality and the outcomes. For instance, the public felt the more severe the medical dispute, the more the hospital needs to shoulder the responsibility, regardless of the responsible attribution, which is shared widely among citizens with lower social status. To some extent, the revitalization of the mediation institutions converged the morality and legal rules in dispute resolution. The more efficacy and successful outcomes they received in the dispute resolution process, the more positive attitudes they held toward the system. It would make the mediation committees still under the shadow of the populist pressure. The mediation channels have to cater to, rather than reshape perception of justice among ordinary citizens.

Finally, the bargained authoritarianism commodified the state-society relations. As the data and interviews showed, the resolution process has become an economic bargaining meeting with bidding for prices. The institutional design of the mediation channel shifted the citizen's right-related discourses to the economic bargaining process, which also neutralized the right pursuits of the citizens, and commercialized the state-society relations.

5.5 Summary

According to the Han Feizi (Chen, 2000), "If those who have no merit are rewarded, the fortunes will be ruined, and the popularity of the people will be lost." Han Feizi emphasized the promotion of consistent institutional responses to punishment and rewards which was essential to promote the legitimacy of the governance. In practice, however, over-compensating or buying stability is widely applied as a pragmatic response to dispute resolution. This chapter examines the mechanism of buying stability by analyzing the compensation distribution in medical disputes resolutions. This form of strategy has not yet been systematically studied due to either data limits or inconsistent responses among various types of social disputes (Davenport, 2005). This chapter aims to fill this vein. Drawing on quantitative and qualitative evidence, this chapter shows that distributive justice, political concerns, as well as economic reasons shaped the outcomes of compensation distribution. On the distributive justice perspective, through the mediation channels, disputes that involve severe medical results are more likely to receive larger compensation to satisfy the public perception of justice and morality. It reflected the combination of law and morality in the distribution process, as all decisions are rule-binding or in accordance with the formal procedures. The compensation distribution outcomes also favored persistent disputants who are considered as troublemakers to prevent disruptive actions and restore social order. Within the mediation channel, economic concern is also crucial element in dispute resolution. The mediation committees have effectively transformed itself into an effective tool in dispute resolution as well as bargaining channel to settle monetary claims in exchange for peace.

Buying stability is a common tool of social management. The government consciously apply buying stability as an approach to shifting citizens' focus on right protection to economic bargaining to neutralize the nature of the dispute. However, the frequent use of "carrots" to deter the activists may also increase the political space to encourage more disruptive actions and commodify the state—society relations. To avoid the inefficacy and negative effects of buying stability, the government has increasingly shifted the role of compensation distribution to the centralized mediation channel—People's Mediation. It finds that the aim of the government-sponsored centralized bargaining channel is to act as a preventive repression strategy to manage social disputes prior its escalation into collective actions or mass incidents. Through the distribution of compensation based on both rules and discretion, the government could prevent the escalation of social disputes without resorting to forceful repression.

The People's Mediation preformed the role of the centralized bargaining channel. The aim of the centralized bargaining channel shoulders the dual goal of addressing compensation claims and settling social disputes. On the one hand, it performs as an alternative legal channel to make judgements based on facts; on the other hand, it applies discretion to make concessions to patients based on informal rules. Through the centralized bargaining channel, the mediation committee responds to patients' grievances and redirects them towards the economic bargaining process under its guidance. More specifically, the mechanism pays special attention to the potential persistent disputants who are considered as troublemakers and make concessions to this group of patients. This study finds that managing medical disputes in China involves more than merely seeking medical facts; it involves a combination of economic bargaining and preventing the occurrence of social disturbances. The government-sponsored centralized bargaining channel further politicizes the medical dispute mediation process.

More importantly, this study finds that diversified strategies were applied to manage small- and large-scale compensation cases. The mediators have adopted informal rules such as "divide and control" to pay special attention to sensitive cases involving more severe medical outcomes and large compensation claims. Davenport (2007) asserted that disaggregation is specifically useful if we expect the government to respond to different challenges with distinct repressive strategies. Government is becoming more sophisticated and experienced by applying various coping strategies, either "carrots or sticks," in addressing disputes. It has attempted to balance organizational interests, as well as satisfy compensation claims, by developing various coping strategies.

Beyond its substantive findings, this chapter also revisits patient-doctor relationships in China. The bargaining process has further deteriorated and commercialized patient-doctor relationships, rendering the trust-building process between the two sides more difficult. On the other hand, social disputes among patients and hospitals are also politicized, and the fundamental deficiencies in the public health system remain as they are. The dispute resolution was inevitably intertwined with the political concerns of maintaining social stability and redressing personnel grievances since the compensation distribution outcome was jointly shaped by patients' tactics and resources owned by hospitals. Therefore, underlying conflicts and compromises between hospitals and the local government are more evident and continue to exist.

Commercialized doctor-patient relationships also tie the hands of the hospitals and cause them to be selective by cherry-picking patients. For instance, during the fieldwork, some doctors commented,

> The patients sometimes did not trust us. After these years, I am aware to protect my own rights. I think I can identify the difficult patients based on my experiences. Make sure you have explained the risks of the medical treatment to the patients and made them signed on the consent form. Don't take risky moves if the patients and their family members do not trust you.[17]

It is necessary to recognize the limitations of this empirical finding. First, this study was based on a small data set of medical disputes and used only the results of compensations to "quantify" the extent to which medical disputes were resolved, which may have oversimplified the issue because grievances may not be measured

[17] Interview with the doctor in one tertiary hospital February 2017.

by money only. Second, this study did not aim to identify the relationship between compensation and the occurrence of collective actions because in reality, the disruptive tactics used to harass hospitals rarely occurred. In this Chapter, I assessed the factors shaping their decisions and causes of variations among uneven compensation distribution. Further studies could contribute to examining the relationship between the application of mediation institutions and the occurrence of collective actions directly. Third, due to data limitations, the findings could be generalized only to social disputes between individuals and organizations. More systematic or comparative studies could contribute to an understanding of dispute resolution politics in China. However, using medical disputes as a proxy explains the conflicting goals of the government and its delegated institutions in promoting a new style of buying stability.

Through the empirical studies, the main body of the book examines the government's coping strategy towards noncompliance behaviors and how the government incorporates and prevents the repeated occurrence of collective actions by reintroducing the institutional channel to absorb the personal grievance. The authorities have established an all-encompassing stability maintenance system to re-choir all necessary political authorities to prevent the occurrence of social disruptions, centring around of the mediation institutions. By doing so, it politicized the social dispute resolution process but also commodified the state—society relations, dampened the rule of law, and failed to promote better patient-doctor relations. Next, the conclusion chapter summarizes the overall findings, limitations and potential contributions of this book.

References

Amengual, M. (2018) Buying stability: The distributive outcomes of private politics in the Bolivian mining industry. *World Development, 104*: 31–45.

Benney, J. (2016) Weiwen at the Grassroots: China's stability maintenance apparatus as a means of conflict resolution. *Journal of Contemporary China, 25*(99): 389–405.

Cai, Y. (2005) China's moderate middle class: the case of homeowners' resistance. *Asian Survey, 45*(5): 777–799.

Chen, Qiyou. 2000. "Han Fei Zi xin jiaozhu" ("Han Feizi, with new collations and commentary") (Shanghai Classics Publishing House).

Chen, X. (2009) The power of "troublemaking": protest tactics and their efficacy in China. *Comparative Politics, 41*(4): 451–471.

Chen, X. (2012) *Social protest and contentious authoritarianism in China.* Cambridge University Press.

Chen, Z. (2009) Launch of the health-care reform plan in China. *The Lancet, 373*(9672), 1322–1324.

Chen, J., & Zhang, Q. (2019) "Difang zhengfu chuli shehui maodun de "fenjiyingdui" jizhi fenxi—yi S sheng M shi yiliaojiufen weili" ("Local government's graduated control mechanism in handling social disputes: case of medical disputes in M city S province") (Public Administration Review) in Chinese, 12(3): 85–103.

Cunningham, K. G., Dahl, M., & Frugé, A. (2017) Strategies of resistance: Diversification and diffusion. *American Journal of Political Science, 61*(3): 591–605.

Davenport, C. (2005) Understanding covert repressive action: The case of the US government against the Republic of New Africa. *Journal of Conflict Resolution, 49*(1), 120–140.

Davenport, C. (2007) State repression and political order. *Annual Review of Political Science, 10*(1): 1–23.

Earl, J. (2003) Tanks, tear gas, and taxes: Toward a theory of movement repression. *Sociological theory, 21*(1): 44–68.

Earl, J. (2011) Political repression: Iron fists, velvet gloves, and diffuse control. *Annual review of sociology, 37*: 261–284.

Earl, J. (2004) Controlling protest: New directions for research on the social control of protest in Authority in Contention (Research in Social Movements, Conflicts and Change, Vol. 25), edited by Myers, D.J. and Cress, D.M., Emerald Group Publishing Limited: 55–83.

Edwards, B., & McCarthy, J. D. (2004) Resources and social movement mobilization. *The Blackwell companion to social movements*:116–152.

Eggleston, K., Lu, M., Li, C., Wang, J., Yang, Z., Zhang, J., & Quan, H. (2010). Comparing public and private hospitals in China: Evidence from Guangdong. *BMC Health Services Research, 10*: 1–11.

Feng. Y, & Cao, Q. (2014) Popularised Judiciary in Rural China: Paternalistic Approaches and Enchanted Legal Consciousness. *Hong Kong LJ, 44*: 651–675.

Fu, D. (2017) Disguised collective action in China. *Comparative Political Studies, 50*(4): 499–527.

Gallagher, M. E., & Wang, Y. (2011) Users and non-users: Legal experience and its effect on legal consciousness. In *Chinese justice: civil dispute resolution in contemporary China*, edited by Woo, M. Y., & Gallagher, M. E., Cambridge University Press, 204–233.

Hadfield, G. K. (2008) Framing the choice between cash and the courthouse: Experiences with the 9/11 Victim Compensation Fund. *Law & Society Review, 42*(3): 645–682.

Halegua, A. (2008) Getting paid: Processing the labor disputes of China's migrant workers. Berkeley *J. Int'l L., 26*: 254–322.

He, X., & Feng, J. (2021) Unfamiliarity and Procedural Justice: Litigants' Attitudes Toward Civil Justice in Southern China. *Law & Society Review, 55*(1): 104–138.

He, X. (2021) Divorce in China. In *Divorce in China*. New York University Press.

Hinterleitner, M. (2017) Reconciling perspectives on blame avoidance behaviour. *Political Studies Review, 15*(2): 243–254.

Hu, J. (2011) Grand mediation in China. *Asian Survey, 51*(6): 1065–1089.

Hu, J., & Zhang, X. (2023) Digital Governance in China: Dispute Settlement and Stability Maintenance in the Digital Age, Journal of Contemporary China, https://doi.org/10.1080/10670564.2023.2261877.

Huang, P. C. (2005) Divorce law practices and the origins, myths, and realities of judicial "mediation" in China. *Modern China, 31*(2): 151–203.

Lee, C. K., & Zhang, Y. (2013) The power of instability: Unraveling the microfoundations of bargained authoritarianism in China. *American journal of sociology, 118*(6): 1475–1508.

McCarthy, J. D., Britt, D. W., & Wolfson, M. (1991) The institutional channeling of social movements by the state in the United States. *Research in social movements, conflicts and change, 13*(2): 45–76.

Michelson, E. (2007) Climbing the dispute pagoda: grievances and appeals to the official justice system in rural China. *American sociological review, 72*(3): 459–485.

Noakes, J., & Gillham, P. (2007) Police and protester innovation since Seattle. *Mobilization: an international quarterly, 12*(4): 335–340.

O'Brien, K. J., & Li, L. (2006) *Rightful resistance in rural China*: Cambridge University Press.

Schock, K. (2013) The practice and study of civil resistance. *Journal of Peace Research, 50*(3): 277–290.

Siminato, A. (2020) "Harmony"(HE 和) and "Coherence"(LI 理) in Neo-Confucianism. *Journal of East-West Thought, 2*(10): 103–118.

Su, Y., & He, X. (2010) Street as courtroom: State accommodation of labor protest in South China. *Law & Society Review, 44*(1): 157–184.

Tsai, L. L. (2015) Constructive Noncompliance. *Comparative politics, 47*(3): 253–279.
Tong, Z. (2014) Practical Moral Consciousness in Rights Claims: Petition Letters on Chinese Village Elections *Rural China, 11*(1), 1–45. https://brill.com/view/journals/rchs/11/1/article-p1_1.xml.
Yusupova, G. (2022) How does the politics of fear in Russia Work? The case of social mobilisation in support of minority languages. *Europe-Asia Studies, 74*(4): 620–641.
Zhang, J., & Cai, Y. (2019) Medical disputes and mediation in China: Government and responsibility shifting. *China Information, 33*(3): 350–371.
Zhuang, W., & Chen, F. (2015) "Mediate First": The revival of mediation in labour dispute resolution in China. *The China Quarterly, 222*: 380–402.

Chapter 6
Conclusion

千丈之堤，溃于蚁穴。
A little leak will sink a great ship.
—韩非子Han Feizi《喻老》*[Illustrations of Laozi's Teachings]*

This book examines how the law, political concerns, and social factors jointly shape China's politicized medical dispute resolution process. This concluding chapter revisits how patients', mediators', and doctors' lives are connected through medical dispute resolution. It concludes and summarizes the key findings of the previous chapters, their theoretical implications, and the book's limitations. The politicization of medical dispute resolution involves the politicization of issues, institutions, and the dispute resolution process and its outcomes. By doing so, it discourages potential collective actions and shifts disputants' focus from rights- and law-related concerns to monetary claims. This chapter suggests that the politicization of social dispute resolution may maintain social stability but does so at the longer-term cost of commercializing patient-doctor relations, eroding social trust, and endangering the foundation of the rule of law.

6.1 Overview

The Chinese government has become adept at sophisticatedly managing social disputes and maintaining social stability through noncoercive and preventive strategies. This book examines the politicized medical dispute resolution in contemporary China, where controversial medical disputes have prompted governments to apply institutional responses to curtail hospital disturbances and maintain social stability at the grassroots. It systematically studies evolving medical dispute resolution institutions and contributes to our understanding of contemporary China's politicized social dispute resolution process.

First, this book places the medical dispute resolution discussion in the political field. It reviews the theoretical and institutional adaptation of dispute resolution

J. Wu, *Politicized Medical Dispute Resolution in China*, Understanding China,
https://doi.org/10.1007/978-981-97-6961-2_6

institutions in China and traces the historical changes in medical dispute resolution since the 1980s. It reflects the Chinese government's continuous efforts to adapt to the changing environment to sustain good governance and be responsive to disputants. It advances scholarly understanding of the changing and evolving institutional responses towards social disputes and the revival of People's Mediation institutions in the 2010s. It also proposes a framework for understanding the institutional foundation of people's mediation, which was based on the complex interaction between the rule of law, social power, and stability maintenance concerns.

Next, this book examines the recent phenomena of hospital violence in China. Existing scholarship attributes hospital disturbances to patient-doctor distrust, health disparities, and cultural factors. In this book, I investigate the rise of hospital violence from a rightful resistance perspective and trace government curtailment of such law-breaking behaviors, impelled by moral indignation and social stability maintenance concerns. Based on a case pool drawn from media archives, I find that the citizens have adopted noncompliance behaviors to advance their interests and hold the local government accountable. I also find that the criminalization of hospital violence has encountered selective punishment-style law enforcement at the street level, often contingent upon the disputants' moral power, the level of their disruptive actions, and the severity of the outcome. The selective punishment resulting from fragmented institutional responses and conflicting inter-agency interests have given rise to hospital violence and led to hospitals adopting self-protection strategies, further deteriorating doctor-patient relations. It also exposed the inefficacy of formal institutions in dispute resolution. The increasing controversy over hospital violence has polarized public discord and anger, prompting the Chinese government to shift from legal responses to mediation channels in addressing social disputes.

The book then examines the responses of People's Mediation institutions, as alternatives to inefficient legal institutions, to address bottom-up grievances. People's mediation has been increasingly politicized due to all-compassing stability maintenance schemes and the salience of social disputes. How do politicized mediation institutions absorb popular grievances? I explain how mediation is carried out, investigate mediators' sophisticated toolkits and diversified strategies, and show how they contribute to mediation institutions' success and efficacy. Through intensive fieldwork, I find that mediators' political and social embeddedness make them suitable intermediaries between public institutions and citizens to overcome power asymmetries. Through their bridging role, mediators achieve multiple goals, including providing psychological comfort to disputants, discouraging potential collective actions to maintain social stability, and facilitating compensation distribution to shift citizens' rights-related concerns into monetary claims. From a comparative perspective, this book helps researchers understand how government-embedded mediation institutions shape dispute resolution from a comparative perspective through the case of China. It also advanced scholarly understanding of state-society relations in the new era by investigating the government's continuous efforts to remake the third realm in China.

Today, many social disputes are derived from citizens' materialistic and non-civic claims (Chen, 2020). Providing monetary compensation to disputants has become a common practice to settle conflicts, as failing to address the monetary compensation issue could easily trigger collective actions. To better understand the bargaining process between citizens and public institutions, I propose a framework that examines the rationale for compensation distribution through the People's Mediation committees. I find that political concern, distributive justice, and economic cost concerns jointly determine the compensation claims decisions through mediation channels. Mediation channels enhanced stability maintenance schemes by promoting consistent distribution practices and remaining flexible to respond to citizens' grievances.

Generally speaking, this book provides a detailed analysis of the political responses to medical disputes through a mixed-method and interdisciplinary approach. Medical disputes, especially hospital violence, have created disruptions in hospitals and imposed uncertainty in social governance and stability maintenance. Political stability concerns and government interests have essentially rewritten doctor-patient relationships and led to the politicization of medical disputes. Dispute resolution is based on neither medical factors drawn from professional judgements nor legal rules but complex interactions between political, legal, and social factors. To realize multiple and sometimes conflicting goals, the politicization of medical dispute resolution depends on quasi-government institutions, People's Mediation Committees, undermining the possibility of collective action and playing a central role in shaping the dispute resolution process, decision-making, and outcomes. This book enables us to understand medical dispute resolution in China and provides a new lens to examine all-encompassing social stability maintenance schemes and institutional responses to social dispute resolution.

6.2 Patients, Doctors, and Mediators

This book examines why medical disputes have become prevalent in China and the government's politicized responses. Politicization is a process that makes (social) issues part of politics (de Wilde, 2011; Bolsen & Druckman, 2015). The government politicized the medical dispute resolution process to respond to citizens' grievances, address social disputes, and maintain social order. The politicization had two sources—the norms conflict between scientific medical knowledge, laymen's grievances, and public perceptions of distributive justice, and the conflict between the public's heightened rights consciousness and the government's increasing social stability demands.

The information asymmetry and mistrust between doctors and patients have resulted in perceptions of injustice and inefficiency in the medical dispute resolution process. Patients sometimes apply disruptive actions to protect their interests, contradicting the government's social stability maintenance priority. This dilemma prompted government intervention in professional and private spheres to resolve grievances and find justice for disputant parties. The politicization of dispute resolution redefined the nature of medical disputes and extended the medical dispute resolution process beyond the professional arena by incorporating political and social concerns and drawing in new actors. Because of the controversial and salient nature of medical disputes, politicizing the resolution promoted mediators to perform as informal state agents to balance the interests of hospitals and patients. Thus, patients', mediators', and doctors' lives are connected through medical dispute resolution.

In the late 1980s, China's public health system entered a market-based era (Hsiao, 1995). As the central government has decreased the financial support to the health system, it has changed the public health system in China in two ways. First, the removal of the referral system incentivized patients to the higher-tier hospitals that are usually located in a few megacities (Eggleston et al., 2008; Yao, 2016; Liu and Hsiao, 1995), which led to the Mathew effect and the imbalance in health resources distribution. Second, the public health system in China has embraced commercial logic to make ends meet by engaging in outsourcing and privatization, changing the nature of doctor-patient relations. The public image of healthcare professionals is deteriorating and becoming stigmatized. Scholars and observers have widely reported and examined hospital corruption, including red packets (a form of disreputable monetary exchange between patients and doctors) and bonuses or kickbacks from pharmaceutical companies (Guo and Xu, 2022). Increased out-of-pocket health spending and concerns about "amoral" medical workers have made patients place high demands and expectations on doctors, further deteriorating patient-doctor relations.

As such, patients' grievances, anger, and penchant for disruptive actions lie close to the surface. Since the 2000s, citizens' increased rights- and legal-consciousness have prompted them to protect their rights vigorously (Li, Liu and O'Brien, 2012). When existing institutionalized channels fail to address their pursuits, they quickly shift their target to local government or apply disruptive or collective actions to make themselves heard. Likewise, hospital violence, as disruptive actions, takes place due to failures to address medical disputes. Due to social stability maintenance concerns, the government often grants leniency and compensation to avoid escalating disputes, signaling the possibility of government "concessions" towards patients' moral-economic claims. Frequent media reports of hospital violence and government concessions have reshaped patients' perceptions of cost-efficient actions, motivating many to apply disruptive actions to hold hospitals accountable. Changes in China's political opportunity structure have motivated more patients to resort to disruptive actions to protect their rights or pursue economic claims, taking advantage of the hospitals' and government's conflicting interests. Lacking autonomous and professional organizations, patients found it hard to resort to patient advocacy groups or alliances to protect their rights, but chose collective actions as an alternative. Their right-protection and petitioning activity was often atomized and scattered, which also limited their perceived risks from the government perspective. In other words, patients also proactively politicized their medical disputes to gain mass/public support and spark government intervention to accelerate the dispute resolution process.

At the other end of the spectrum, doctors, suffering from high workload, a lack of respect, and limited professional autonomy (Yao, 2019), have become scapegoats for China's inefficient health system. In 2009, Chinese authorities launched a new health reform program by re-introducing primary health services at the community level. The initiative aimed to ease the workloads of health professionals in higher-tier hospitals by promoting service at the grassroots. However, upper-level-healthcare-seeking behaviors persisted among patients, given the uneven professional qualifications among healthcare professionals in China. For instance, in 2014, according to the National Health and Planning Committees, around fifty percent of licenced doctors at grassroots (primary) health institutions did not have a bachelor's or higher educational qualification (Yao, 2016). The disparities among healthcare professionals and uneven development across regions are root causes of medical disputes. Non-local residents often seek medical help and second opinions in large cities due to China's imbalanced health resource distribution, leaving tertiary hospitals packed with patients daily. Doctors at tertiary hospitals must see at least 100 patients daily, twice as many as doctors in the US. Per Arthur Kleinman (2015), the average meeting time with a single patient dropped to two minutes, making necessary eye contact and caregiving impossible and establishing trust and building affection between doctors and patients harder. Holding high expectations towards hospitals, frustrated patients become even angrier when outcomes are displeasing, with some turning their grievances into violence. However, health workers' voices or professionals opinions are largely absent from the discourse.

In addition to their professional roles, healthcare professionals now take on politicized roles. Constrained by their institutional identities and public embeddedness (Yao, 2015), healthcare professionals are also under tight state control, facing pressure from government authorities. Healthcare professionals belonged to the all-companssing social stability maintenance system and needed to bow to the political pressure. As Benjamin Liebman (2016) illustrated, hospitals operate under the shadow of popular justice and social stability maintenance goals. Healthcare professionals and hospital representatives cannot rely on professional knowledge to keep the peace; they also face political pressure to compromise or selectively intervene to calm disputants and discourage collective actions. The history of the health system in China is the history of public hospital development and changing relations between the Party and professionals. Public hospitals have long been considered public institutions as they are government-financed and must align with the government in preventing and addressing disputes. However, the goal of social stability may endanger medical professionals' authority and reduce their dignity and vocational safety.

Local government's hands are often tied when dealing with medical disputes, reflecting China's governance dilemma. Some reform measures have improved hospital security and prevented hospital violence, including criminalizing hospital violence, changing media attitudes towards hospital violence to reshape citizens' cost-efficient perspectives, and, in particular, revitalizing public mediation institutions for medical dispute resolution. China's officials cannot fully rely on legal channels and formal rules to address social problems; thus, the government now relies on mediators to resolve medical disputes and make tradeoffs between patients and hospitals, strategically combining formal and informal rules flexibly to achieve social stability and relieve bottom-up grievances. Mediators have become an intermediary belt bridging the government and its citizens. Per Lubman (1967), mediators have been China's primary dispute resolution model since the Mao era, shouldering the social goals of maintaining and regulating harmonious social relations and the political role of popularizing policy to enhance the government's grassroots legitimacy.

The gratitude letter from the patient (Fig. 6.1) revealed how the mediators help to communicate on behalf of the patient to reach a reconciliation in dispute resolution. The mediator was praised highly by the patient for his active, patience and devotion to the mediation process. After the mediation, the patient even wanted to provide a red pocket to the mediators, which was of course rejected by the mediator. During the fieldwork, many mediators told the author that they took the job not because of the monetary incentives, but want to do something for social governance even after retirement. "My retirement salary is high enough to make a good living (around 10,000 yuan). The allowance for me is just a symbolic reward."[1] The unsalaried mediators helped to relieve and free the local government from heavy investment and involvement in social governance in a cost-efficient manner.

Unlike the public sphere that declared autonomous from and prior to the state in the western society and could express and publicize their opinions freely (Somers, 1995; Habermas, 1991; Wakeman, 1993), the intermediary realm between state and society in China is not autonomous, but under the government influence and sponsorship. Like minimalist governance (Huang, 2019), the Chinese government does not always rely on the Weberian bureaucracy to realize its rule, instead, it relies on the semi-officials such as mediators to regulate social relations at the grassroots and achieve social control. Mediators are often government officials or professionals deeply embedded in the social and political system; like the social gentry, they link officialdom and ordinary citizens. On the one hand, mediators are under moral pressure to protect the interests of vulnerable disputants. Their authority, personal relations, and *guanxi* could easily win disputants' respect and trust and help them negotiate from an advantaged position with hospitals, which have more and better resources. These informal institutions, existing and operating outside official channels (Helmke & Levitsy, 2004), can flexibly promote reconciliation, changing disputants' mindsets through persuasion, affective strategies, law popularizing, etc. On the other hand, the government trusts mediators due to their political embeddedness, relying on them to achieve its social governance goals and maintain its authority. Mediators can flexibly diffuse government preferences through their mediation process without resorting to coercive power, achieving goals of social governance more effectively.

Today, mediators have been revived and adapted to address new social disputes and new governance aims by growing professionalism. Taking advantage of their semi-official identity, mediators can better respond to disputants' emotional demands to manage and relieve citizens' grievances. They can also bridge the cognitive gaps between laymen and professionals through legal popularization and persuasion. In

[1] Interview with a senior mediator in September 2017.

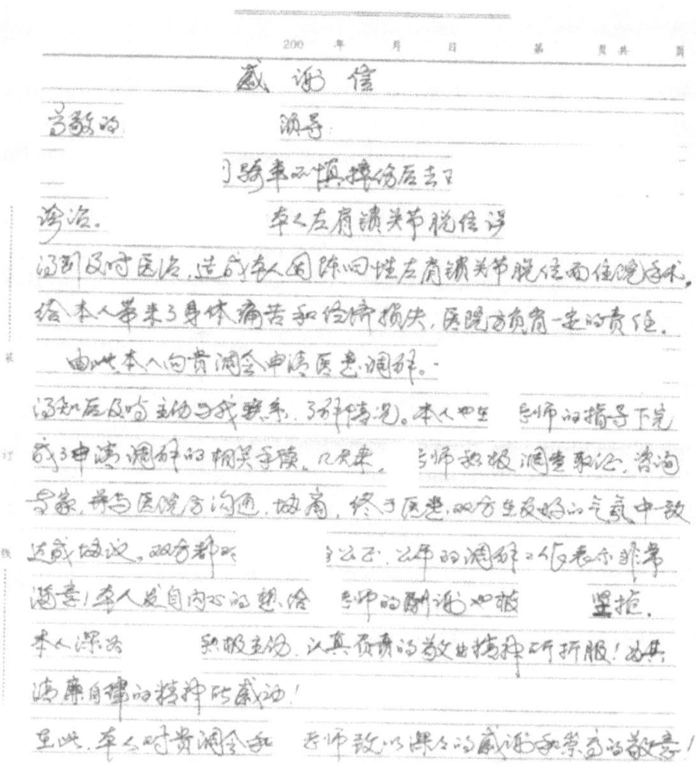
200 年 月 日 第 页 共 页

感谢信

尊敬的 领导：

因骑车不慎摔伤后去

诊治。 本人左肩锁关节脱位未

得到及时医治，造成本人因陈旧性左肩锁关节脱位而住院手术。

给本人带来了身体痛苦和经济损失，医院方负有一定的责任。

由此本人向贵调委会申请医患调解。

得知后及时主动与我联系，了解情况。本人也在 老师的指导下完

成了申请调解的相关手续。几天来， 老师积极调查取证，咨询

专家，并与医院方沟通、协商，终于医患双方在友好的气氛中一致

达成协议。双方都对 办公室、老师的调解工作表示非常

满意！本人发自内心的想，给 老师的酬谢也被 婉拒。

本人深为 积极主动、认真负责的敬业精神所折服！为其

清廉自律的精神所感动！

在此，本人对贵调委会和 老师致以深深的感谢和崇高的敬意！

Fig. 6.1 Gratitude letter from disputant

dealing with disputes, they can flexibly combine logical, legal, and political principles to prevent dispute escalation, striking a subtle balance between top-down political pressure to maintain social stability and bottom-up populist pressure to demonstrate and relieve grievances.

6.3 Politicized Social Disputes Resolution

Unlike in Western regimes, where social disputes are defined as private sphere conflicts, social dispute resolution in China often requires government intervention. The ideal state-society relations authorities seek to realize in China involves maintaining social stability while building a harmonious society with sound social relationships. Failing to address social disputes would arouse moral indignation towards the authorities' failure to follow the Party's mass-line strategy and perform the people's will, possibly endangering social stability and the Party's legitimacy. The politicization of social dispute resolution takes place in a contentious environment. The high salience of social disputes has prompted the government to deal with the resulting tensions cautiously. Social dispute resolution has become part of politics in China, and its associated processes and results have been politicized.

In ancient China, imperial governments refrained from directly engaging in social dispute resolution unless necessary. Due to the illegibility and the state's weak capacity, many social disputes were reconciled via the local social gentry, who had accumulated knowledge, land, and authority. While this division between the civil and the state was common (Fei, 1980), the rise of the modern state and China's powerful Party-state system changed the laissez-faire status quo. Beginning in 1949, the work-unit system reorganized society in an ordered and disciplined way, sweeping away many autonomous and civic intermediaries (e.g., business associations) in Chinese society (Ma, 2002) and becoming the intermediary between the citizen and the government. The work unit system shouldered various "government" roles as a government agent (Zhang, 2016), including dossier management, marriage approval, and dispute resolution, brokering the loose citizen-government relationship.

Since the 1980s, rapid economic growth and political change have led to earth-shaking social development and brought new social problems. The closing years of the twentieth and the early years of the twenty-first centuries witnessed the politicization of dispute resolution, as citizens increasingly organized and frequently adopted collective actions to protect their rights. Removing the work-unit system as an intermediary has forced the government to face and deal with bottom-up grievances directly. Although social disputes occur between civic actors and are considered less regime-threatening, government officials are keenly aware of the political difficulties of addressing such social disputes, especially between citizens and public or private institutions, and must make tradeoffs between the parties. The situation became more difficult as citizens frequently applied rightful resistance to prioritize their claims, potentially endangering social stability and the government's legitimacy. Satisfying all bottom-up claims would dampen local economic development and encourage collective actions. Hence, local government sometimes behaved in ways that enhanced its legitimacy and reputation for protecting citizens' rights, responding to their claims and appearing concerned about their organized actions and perceptions of the government. On the other hand, local governments also aligned with the interests of private or public institutions, for economic reasons.

Because of their heavy political and economic burden, local governments began to rely on other institutions to rebuild the intermediary link between it and disputants by channeling disputants into authorized channels—including the letter and visit bureau, legal channels, and the semi-formal people's mediation institutions discussed in this book—thereby politicizing People's Mediation institutions, medical disputes, and the dispute resolution process and outcomes.

First, politicized social issues. Increasing controversy and pluralized actors have accelerated social disputes' politicization. From the government's perspective, social disputes carry the possibility of creating social disturbances and reducing Chinese authorities' legitimacy. Failing to address social disputes would expose institutional inertia and inefficacy. Meanwhile, social issues have become more complex by drawing various social and political players into the process. For instance, a social dispute is a conflict involving the bargain between citizens and public or private institutions, involving legal and public security and administrative forces. The expansion of involved actors (De Wilde, Leupold, and Schmidtke, 2016) has made conflicts more visible, urgent, unavoidable, and no longer confined to the private sphere, making government intervention and politicization inevitable.

The consequences of politicizing medical disputes could be two-fold. On the one hand, it undermines the authority of professional norms and increases levels of distrust. When medical disputes are politicized, involved patients and families face greater exposure to uncertainty and asymmetric power relations between patients and doctors and public institutions, casting doubt on the dispute resolution process and creating distrust towards in health institutions. On the other hand, politicization also provides ordinary citizens the political space to hold doctors, hospitals, and local government accountable. Since the government prioritizes political stability maintenance, citizens could (threaten to) apply disruptive actions to advance their interests.

Second, politicizing social disputes also politicizes institutions, as People's Mediation institutions have been responsible for social dispute resolution since 2010, redirecting personal grievances and the government's responses. Fairly speaking, mediation committees are government-embedded dispute resolution institutions, a crucial element of China's social stability maintenance system. Though often disguised as a "third party" system, satisfying the state's grassroots stability goal remains the institutions' ultimate political goal. However, interestingly, the politicized mediation channel also involvd an array of de-politicized strategies to shift the nature of conflict from rightful resistance to economic bargaining and discourage popular involvement in disputes. To achieve this goal, local governments mobilize various groups of semi-officials to restore the third realm by playing various roles, including working as social workers to provide psychological effort, as government spokespersons to prevent disruptive actions, and as legal workers to popularize regulations and laws. For instance, these semi-officials usually resorted to moralist discourse and affective strategies to persuade the disputants. Such depoliticization approaches accelerate and smooth the dispute resolution process, avoiding agitating the disputants. Depoliticization and politicization strategies complement each other and enhance the efficacy of People's Mediation committees in dispute resolution.

Third, dispute resolution processes and outcomes are also politicized. The mediation process is full of social power interaction and political persuasion, and its outcomes are based on concerns about social stability, governance, and political rules. The mediation process is not devoid of political and social pressure for citizens or hospitals. For instance, disputants, especially those with limited social and political resources, may be under psychological, social, and political pressure to accept dispute resolution results. Professionals may also need to compromise in medical disputes to avoid responsibility or reach a speedy resolution. Political first principles may not always align with either disputants' interests. Since mediators are deeply embedded within the political system, they inevitably align government interests to address disputes efficiently, puts disputants' interests at risk.

There are three critical aspects in dealing with social disputes. The first is asymmetric power relations. Unlike courts, mediators rely on social institutions (face, social networks, emotional work, etc.) to address disputes. In most mediated cases, mediators address the asymmetric power relations between vulnerable citizens and "powerful" institutions to empower citizens. Mediation institutions use not only the language of rules and law, but the language of morality and favor to show benevolence and compassion to disputants. As Chaps. 4 and 5 showed, the medical dispute resolution process in China is not devoid of social and political power and shoulders the dual responsibility of addressing social disputes and avoiding irritating the public by reflecting moral principles. Vulnerable and pitiable citizens are often favored in the process under benevolent moral principles.

The second involves disruptive actions. The past two decades have witnessed a rise in rightful resistance and collective actions, particularly in social disputes, leading the government to adopt covert preventive strategy to maintain social stability. Mediators must take these "troublemakers" seriously and flexibly resort to political deterrence through cooperation with other coercive institutions to maintain social stability and de-legitimate their disruptive actions.

The third factor concerns inherent consistency and selective intervention. Mediation becomes a centralized compensation bargaining system for dispute resolution. It promotes consistent institutionalized outcomes by standardizing compensation distribution principles to ease economic costs, while creating exceptions in a case-by-case fashion to flexibly address disputes.

6.4 Bargaining-Style Mediation

In recent decades, political considerations have been introduced into many areas of society (Bourdieu, 1991). For instance, social dispute resolution institutions are applied as a political tool. This book examines an old-yet-new institution—people's mediation channel—and investigates how mediators address medical disputes and factors influence dispute resolution outcomes. I find that embedded political goals and interlocked personal authority and relations have provided formal and informal institutional foundations for the mediation channel, promoting mediators to selectively compromise legal rules to satisfy social and political goals to maintain social stability. Through the mediation channel, economic bargaining decisions are a joint outcome of distributive justice, social stability priority, and economic concerns, reflecting the mediation channel's institutional development by balancing various goals.

Mediation institutions' political embeddedness differentiates Chinese-style mediation from other types. People's Mediation institutions were once an institutional innovation for dealing with social disputes. Dating back to the Shaan'ganning era, Ma Xiwu-style mediation has represented both bottom-up interests and top-down government directions to diffuse new policies and social norms. It helped the Party perpetrate policy, change the cultural atmosphere, and address disputes. In the Mao era, mediation institutions persisted and were embedded within the work-unit and community systems to address various social and civil disputes.

However, the role of mediation declined in the reform and open-up era. With the rise of legal institutions and the accompanying decline of the work-unit system (Zhang, 2016), many mediation institutions reduced their role in representing mass interests, costing them their legitimacy and discursive power in dispute resolution and further diluting the Party's information collection, policy diffusion, and social governance capacities. Mediation could no longer act as a "safety valve" in identifying social disputes in China.

Since the 2010s, mediation institutions have been revitalized and adapted to address emerging social disputes. The introduction of mediation institutions was part of the development of coordinated and integrated stability maintenance institutions, involving relevant departments' coordinated efforts in addressing social disputes. Mediation, taking advantage of its "third-party" status, could de-politicize social disputes, while allowing and enhancing multi-agency collaboration to jointly address disputes in the name of social stability maintenance. Mediation has become the core of the social stability maintenance web, with other departments (police, neighborhood committees, health bureau, etc.) serving as extended networks. As such, the social dispute resolution framework has been supervised by multiple government departments and citizens face a well-knit web of control that prevents disruptive behaviors and relieves grievances through joint efforts.

Mediation institutions have successfully transformed the social conflict resolution process into one of economic bargaining. First, mediation institutions restrain disputants' from applying rights-related framing, de-politizing social conflicts and reducing their politically threatening nature. As widely observed in many medical dispute cases, disputants apply rights-related framing as an open form of resistance to hold hospitals and grassroots states to account. Despite maintaining thousands of connections with government, mediation committees are still considered a "third party" in the dispute resolution process. Taking advantage of their intermediary status, mediators shift disputants away from rights-related discourses to focus on the relevant law, regulations, and precedents.

Second, mediators promote distributive justice to increase personal efficacy in mediation channels. Different from legal channels based on the rule of law, the mediation channel relies on informal rules including morals, *renqing* (favor), face (Hwang, 1987), etc. to make decisions. Mediation committees prioritize moral responsibility to win disputants' hearts, focusing on "outcomes" and personal efficacy rather than procedural justice. Discretion is largely applied, giving "troublemakers" more political attention. By selectively responding to vulnerable citizens' claims, it detaches the mediation process from the power asymmetry and inequality between the disputants and public institutions.

Third, the mediation channel institutionalizes compensation distribution by promoting consistent distribution. The mediation channel is vigilant concerning the side effects of buying stability and refrains from applying the "buying stability" strategy. Mediators utilize personal authority, bureaucratic procedures, and psychological strategies to reshape citizens' compensation expectations, freeing the government from using coercion and lowering the economic costs of social stability maintenance.

Bargaining-style mediation leaves the core of the health system reform untouched but further commercializes the patient-doctor relationship and motivates defensive medicine behaviors (He, 2014) and cherry-picking patients (excluding high-risk patients). It allows the government to ease citizens' grievances efficiently and manage the cost of dispute resolution. However, since the mediation process prioritizes measuring personal efficacy based on compensation outcome, it helps ease grassroots antagonism towards the government but not health institutions. Some Western practices prioritize the importance of apology in mediation (Schneider, 2000; Levi, 1997), whereas many healthcare professionals in China refrain from apologies as they may be used against them as evidence of malpractice. Though many hospital representatives express sorrow and condolences during the mediation process, it has not involved an institutional design aimed at alleviating the mistrust between medical workers and patients. In most cases, the doctor involved does not participate in the mediation process, whether for self-protection or to avoid increasing tensions or agitating the disputant. Patients rely on the doctors' medical proficiency and expect them to satisfy their emotional needs and satisfactions. Medical workers' emotional responses and mediators' affective strategies play crucial roles in dispute resolution. The art of apology has been largely omitted in the current institutional design of mediation institutions.

Meanwhile, bargaining-style mediation has prompted scholars to revisit the role of affective governance in dispute resolution. As discussed in Chap. 4, the success of mediation is attributed to mediators' adopting affective strategies like cooling off, building authority, and building emotional ties to regulate and manage disputants' emotions and psyches to facilitate dispute resolution. As many disputants have heightened emotions or deep grievances, affective strategies could decrease their negative emotions and increase their positive feelings towards the government-embedded mediation committees' efficacy. The approach can also help rewrite the power asymmetry in patient-doctor relations by enabling mediators to leverage disputants' bargaining power. Showing compassion for disputants, especially those in vulnerable positions, could earn mediators their gratitude, reliance, and compliance.

Indeed, China's government has used affective and emotional strategies to maintain social stability and dispute resolution since the revolutionary era. For instance,

Perry (2002) examined how the Party performed "emotion work" to solicit grassroots support and mobilize mass and local elites in land reform. Today, affective strategy persists and has been adapted to settle social disputes between citizens and public institutions. Like father-mother official, meidators contributed to the benevolent governance in China. However, despite aiming to address disputes non-confrontationally, affective strategies may reinforce and reproduce power asymmetry by strengthening the unequal hierarchical relations between citizens, mediators, public institutions, and the local state. To have their concerns addressed, disputants must follow recognized channels and express emotional acquiescence. It not only transformed mediators as skilled emotion worker but also reinforced the power asymmetry between disputants and public institutions.

Third, bargaining-style mediation's efficacy may be fragile and contingent as its success depends on the personal characteristics of disputants and mediators. On the one hand, mediators' capacities and backgrounds are decisive in mediation; their authority and networks could facilitate dispute resolution by pressuring hospitals to accelerate negotiations and allow disputants to accept the compensation distribution outcomes. Local governments form retired officials and new graduates into serviceable mediation committees supervised, organized, and sometimes financed by juridical departments, linking various social classes and developing persuasion in dispute resolution to achieve social management and control goals. Their seniority, capability, and authority may largely contribute to the success of mediation. On the other hand, disputants who lack the resources to address their disputes are more likely to achieve reconciliation through mediation channels. Mediators are intermediaries connecting a target population, especially peripheral social actors with few resources. In comparison, disputants from higher social and economic status are less likely or more difficult to be persuaded through the mediation channels.

Mediation relies on efficient persuasion, psychological efforts, and the mediators' authority. Mediators must bond with disputants to pacify their grievances and channel them to authorized channels, requiring great effort. A lack of authority, personal influence, and networks would make it difficult for mediators to persuade disputants since they would be seen to lack power. Many concerns may arise concerning mediators' capability: Who are qualified mediators? Can they balance the pressure from governments, hospitals, and disputants? Pressure is a mediator's greatest challenge, requiring hours of effort and the constant balancing of conflicting goals and subjects.

6.5 Implications and Limitations of the Study

This book began with a simple puzzle derived from real life: Why do citizens resort to hospital violence to resolve social disputes in China under socialist regime? How does the state respond to social disputes? To answer these questions, this study has examined state-professional-citizen relations in China's politicized medical dispute resolution process since China's reform and opening up.

The Chinese state has traditionally focused on regime-threatening issues, such as organized collective actions pinpointing the political system. However, the regime's survival hinges on social disputes linked to citizens' grievances and interests. As the old saying goes, "A little leak will sink a great ship (千丈之堤，溃于蚁穴)". Thinking beyond occasional, larger-scale collective actions aimed at changing the extant political order and social system, smaller-scale or individualized non-regime threatening actions have increasingly create long-term troubles for rulers. This book has identified the institutionalized patterns of state strategies for dealing with social disputes by absorbing personal grievances, settling unrest through compensation distribution, and preventing dispute escalation.

Throughout the book, I have demonstrated how the complex interactions of moral, political and legal factors shaped the government's response. In dealing with hospital violence cases, the dilemma of maintaining social stability and being responsive to personal grievances affects street-level officials' daily practices. In cases involving small disruptions and disadvantaged citizens, selective punishment or under enforcement of law are widely observed concessions towards personal grievances and blame avoidance. I have also traced the institutional development of mediation committees and mediators' dynamic strategies in negotiating with patients. Empirically, I have examined the logic embedded in the monetary compensation distribution process by considering mediation committees as a centralized bargaining channel to illustrate how moral perceptions of justice, political stability maintenance, and economic concerns have jointly shaped the process and outcomes of medical dispute resolution.

Beyond medical disputes, the institutional foundation of dispute resolution still persisted. In dealing with various types of social disputes (such as labor, and real estate disputes), mediators also need to balance multiple goals of cost efficiency, social stability, and the rule of law collectively. Mediation committees have to adopt a balancing strategy between individual and organized interests. For instance, in dealing with a property crisis, the local government often hold real estate partially accountable to prevent it from bankruptcy, while also protecting the partial interests of the property investors. The balanced approach also reflected the complex goals that the mediation committee pursued. The principle of the rule of law allows the mediation committees to grow organizational professionalism. Yet it doesn't constrain the space for the mediators to maneuver to uphold the regulations flexibly. The political logic reflected the state's persistent stability maintenance mindset. The cost-efficient principle constrained the frequency of applying discretional power and promoted consistency in mediation decisions and protecting the organisational interests of the public institutions. Through the intermediary role of mediation institutions, the Chinese government strike a balance to avoid over and under-responsiveness towards the citizens' grievances.

This book has both theoretical and practical implications for governance and health studies. First, it may prompt us to rethink the autonomy and power of professional groups in China. As the book reveals, prioritizing stability in addressing medical disputes sometimes sacrifices professional organizations' rights to preserve workplace safety and harmony. Since professionals are considered semi-government officials in China, their political embeddedness makes hospitals bow to patients' claims to maintain stability. In this social atmosphere, all public organs involved in stability maintenance have become instruments to maintain social stability at the cost of professional and legal norms. As discussed, politicizing medical dispute resolution may not improve patient-doctor relations, neither prevent the occurrence of medical disputes, but merely a post-up remedy. Though hospital violence has been curtailed, healthcare professionals' insecurities and patients' complaints persist in the health system. The internal crack between professional groups and local government may hinder further health system reform. Countering the trend toward politicization requires efforts from legal and healthcare professionals to build a consensus concerning professionals' enhanced autonomy and development.

A new round of health reform is underway, with the government continuing efforts to regulate healthcare professionals' behaviors and codes of conduct. Most of these measures have remained political or administrative, lacking professional input and consensus concerning disciplining and regulating immoral behavior. Large-scale anti-corruption campaigns have taken place in public hospitals around China to regulate the "dubious" relationship between the pharmaceutical industry and healthcare professionals. Widespread media reports of kickbacks, hospital corruption, and skyrocketing medicine prices[2] have blamed health professionals for China's unsatisfactory health system, further eroding patient-doctor trust.

Interestingly, a recent study by Fu Hongqiao et al. (2023) found that from 2011 to 2018, only 0.4% of out-patients and 1.4% of in-patients provided red packets to medical professionals, a much lower informal payment rate than in other developing countries. However, the public is still more inclined to attribute their health system dissatisfaction to the misconduct of the few corrupt healthcare professionals exposed in the media, a potentially misleading and biased responsible attribution process.

The government's retrenchment has also contributed to the health system's commercialization, a factor neglected in mainstream discourses. Since reforms in the 1990s, hospitals have shouldered a heavy economic burden to finance staff and make ends meet, driving some to engage in profit-making collaborations, including merging, land acquisition, and outsourcing, to sustain their operation. Hospitals have, to some extent, taken the blame for decreasing government resources in the transition era. Moreover, as critical media coverage blooms, distrust towards doctors and the health system may grow. How these policies might affect patient-doctor relations and medical disputes warrants further investigation.

The professional autonomy might be a ultimate solution to medical dispute resolution. Neither the administrative organ nor the mediaiton institutions could effectively supervise and monitor the behaviors of healthcare professionals and prevent the occurrence of medical disputes. It requires a strong professional associations, in addition to the legal channels, to protect the intersts of medical professionals, as well as exercise institutional pressure to dispcline professionals' behaviors to improve the health service quality. These professionals associations could play the dual role

---

[2] See, for instance, Repayment "bypasses" hospitals! Many places cut off the profit chain of medical corruption, http://www.news.cn/politics/2023-08/11/c_1129797632.htm, accessed on September 27, 2023.

of self-protection as well as self-regulation. Politicized medical dispute resolution alone is not sufficient.

Politicized social disputes are not new. For decades, the Chinese government has applied various measures to prevent small-scale social disputes from escalating into large-scale collective actions. In the book, I review the institutional adaptation of mediation committees, adding new functions to accommodate rapid social change and new political demands. This book identifies the institutional foundations of dispute resolution in China, including legal, political and social rules, and how these constraints jointly politicized the social dispute resolution process and its outcomes.

I also demonstrate the limitations of the mediation institution. First, the mediation process is not devoid of influence or power. The mediation system's bureaucratic procedures and mediators' influence and authority may still make disputants compromise and acquiesce. In the face of mediators' expectations and authority, patient disputants are more likely to adjust their expectations and accommodate external willingness, reproducing hierarchical and unequal social relations. Second, the law and rules are inconsistently applied throughout the dispute resolution process. Mediators may prioritize stability maintenance, sacrificing hospitals' interests for social peace. China lacks the medical malpractice law, effective health system, and developed professional norms and autonomy needed to protect the interests of both patients and hospitals. As such, mediation institutions do not improve patient-doctor relations by employing clear-cut dispute resolution criteria, instead reinforcing political stability and social power goals in dispute resolution.

The pan-politicization of social disputes may imply enhanced social control and the government's invisible hand in regulating society. Achieving contradictory goals of the rule of law, social norms, and political stability concerns simultaneously is complicated, and mediation institutions must constantly strive to strike a balance. Strictly following the rules and law may not be compatible with public perceptions of justice and could provoke social grievances and disruptive actions, endangering social stability, while overemphasizing stability maintenance and social norms may conflict with the rule of law and risk "encouraging" citizens' repetitive claims. This is why neither law enforcement nor legal courts could provide satisfactory solutions to social disputes and ceded responsibility towards mediation channels, taking advantage of mediators' complex roles to strike a balance. Mediation committees became centralized bargaining channels for dispute resolution, acting as emotion workers to incentivize both parties to compromise to maintain social management and social control goals.

The continued growth, diversification, and professionalization of the mediation committees are foreseeable as the government longs to pursue social stability; the tradeoff between various conflicting goals may also be sustained. The author wants to draw scholarly and practitioners' attention to the institutionalization of mediation channels by proposing a few policy recommendations. First, mediators' ethical standards are missing from the current politicized dispute resolution framework and must be revisited. With the professionalization of mediation committees, mediators must create a code of conduct to balance potentially conflicting factors, including political stability pressure, disputants' rights, and legal principles. Mediator quality has to be prioritized, and mediators must receive sufficient training to improve their legal and ethical professionalism. As recognized brokers between institutions and citizens, mediators must balance disputants' interests and the government's complex goals. For instance, in addition to raising awareness of their roles and actions, mediators must inform disputants of their positions and possible ethical conflicts. Mediators must be more cautious when pursuing efficiency goals to avoid exerting psychological pressure on disputants and should promote inherent consistency and institutional professionalism by refraining from using their discretionary power. Mediation must protect and prioritize disputants' willingness and understanding.

Second, mediation institutions may be a better medical dispute resolution channel for promoting appropriate apologies and mutual communication between patient and doctor. Promoting appropriate apology and communication procedures could be viewed through a cultural and communication lens rather than from a legal perspective. Candid gestures from involved medical workers are necessary to unknot disputants.

Third, as an official cliché, the urgency of promoting a more efficient health system with qualified healthcare professionals to satisfy citizens' health demands should never be neglected. Promoting earlier diagnoses, affordable health care, and the referral system at the community level and rebuilding healthcare professionals' reputations will always be critical to resolving problems. Transparency in interactions between pharmaceutical companies and hospitals warrants more attention to increase compliance levels in public and private institutions and build patient-doctor trust.

Fourth, medical malpractice law should be enacted, and malpractice and medical negligence standards should be clarified and classified. The existing "regulation on medical malpractice resolution" was promulgated at the administrative level with the dual purposes of addressing medical disputes and justifying administrative sanctions; these dual processes must be separated, as a different logic informs them and could arouse conflicts of interest in professionals reviewing malpractice cases. Overall, the mediation channel should be further professionalized and institutionalized to detach itself from political involvement.

It is also necessary to acknowledge this study's limitations. First, due to limited resources and time, the book's findings were primarily drawn from fieldwork in a single Chinese megacity. Although the leading practices of its People's Mediation Committee and medical dispute resolution process make the fieldwork site a "model city" for other cities, future studies could conduct more comparative research to explore regional variances and study different government-sponsored mediation channels across the nation and their dispute resolution priorities and performance. For instance, in southern coastal areas, folk tradition and local religion (such as *mazu* or *matsu*) have been increasingly incorporated into the mediation practice to enhance its social institutions. Meanwhile, to supplement the fieldwork's limitation, I also drew on cases of hospital violence reported in newspapers and other media streams in various regions; however, online data sources are limited and prone to incompleteness and selection bias, and selective punishment findings may warrant further investigation. In the future, automated text mining could be applied to juridical reports to explore further the causal mechanism between "under-enforcement" and non-compliant behaviors. Future studies could also apply field experiments to test officials' risk perceptions of and responses towards law-breaking behaviors at the street level. Such an approach could contribute to understanding the role of grass-roots law enforcement in stability maintenance and implementing the rule of law in China.

Second, generalizing medical disputes to other social disputes may be constrained. The government's soft-coping and buying-stability strategies could be limited in their potential for generalization to other social disputes. As is typical of social disputes, medical disputes are non-political and non-regime threatening, and their study contributes to understanding how the socialist state politicizes social disputes by redirecting the citizens into institutionalized channels. However, more comparative research could be performed to show the various government strategies for coping with social disputes by categorizing their threat levels. For instance, a comparison between medical and labor disputes would be interesting; a more politically-embedded and organized labor protest may be less likely to draw concessions than a medical dispute. The potential political threats embedded in the different disputes determine the government's response and degree of punishment. Further measuring the degree of threat by differentiating between various types of social disputes may help disclose the government's diversified and incremental coping strategies towards various threats.

Third, this book does not touch upon the causal mechanism between the government's strategy and the occurrences of hospital violence. Through fieldwork, I found that the rise of People's Mediation institutions has absorbed patients' grievances and curtailed hospital violence. However, this leaves room for further research. As an intermediary between the state and its citizens, mediators in China follow their own complex institutional logic in relieving social grievances, and their means of balancing political considerations, legal norms, and social authority may warrant further scholarly attention and empirical tests.

References

Bolsen, T., & Druckman, J. N. (2015) Counteracting the politicization of science. *Journal of Communication*, 65(5): 745–769.

Bourdieu, P. (1991) *Language and symbolic power*. Harvard University Press.

Chen, X. (2020) Civic and Noncivic Activism under Autocracy: Shifting Political Space for Popular Collective Action. *Mobilization: An International Quarterly*, *25*(SI): 623–640.

De Wilde, P. (2011) No polity for old politics? A framework for analyzing the politicization of European integration. *Journal of European integration*, *33*(5): 559–575.

De Wilde, P., Leupold, A., & Schmidtke, H. (2016) Introduction: The differentiated politicisation of European governance. *West European Politics*, *39*(1): 3–22.

Eggleston, K., Ling, L., Qingyue, M., Lindelow, M., & Wagstaff, A. (2008) Health service delivery in China: a literature review. *Health economics*, *17*(2): 149–165.

Fei, X. (1980) *China's gentry: Essays on rural-urban relations*. University of Chicago Press.

Fu, H., Lai, Y., Li, Y., Zhu, Y., & Yip, W. (2023) Understanding medical corruption in China: a mixed-methods study. *Health Policy and Planning, 38*(4): 496–508.

Guo, W., & Xu, B. (2022) Dignity in red envelopes: Disreputable exchange and cultural reproduction of inequality in informal medical payment. *Social Psychology Quarterly, 85*(1): 23–43.

Habermas, J. (1991) The Public Sphere, in Rethinking Popular Culture. C. Mukerji and M. Schudson, University of California Press, 398–404.

He, A. J. (2014) The doctor–patient relationship, defensive medicine and overprescription in Chinese public hospitals: Evidence from a cross-sectional survey in Shenzhen city. *Social science & medicine, 123*: 64–71.

Helmke, G., & Levitsky, S. (2004) Informal institutions and comparative politics: A research agenda. *Perspectives on politics, 2*(4): 725–740.

Hsiao, W. C. (1995) The Chinese health care system: lessons for other nations. *Social science & medicine, 41*(8): 1047–1055.

Huang, P. C. (2019) Rethinking "the Third Sphere": The dualistic unity of state and society in China, past and present. *Modern China, 45*(4): 355–391.

Hwang, K. K. (1987) Face and favor: The Chinese power game. *American journal of Sociology, 92*(4): 944–974.

Kleinman, A. (2015) Care: In search of a health agenda. *The Lancet, 386*(9990): 240–241.

Levi, D. L. (1997) The role of apology in mediation. *NYUL Rev., 72,* 1165.

Li, L., Liu, M., & O'Brien, K. J. (2012) Petitioning Beijing: the high tide of 2003–2006. *The China Quarterly, 210*: 313–334.

Liebman, B. L. (2016) Law in the Shadow of Violence: Can Law Help to Improve Doctor-Patient Trust in China. *Columbia Journal of Asian Law, 30*: 113.

Liu, X., & Hsiao, W. C. (1995) The cost escalation of social health insurance plans in China: its implication for public policy. *Social science & medicine, 41*(8): 1095–1101.

Lubman, S. (1967) Mao and mediation: politics and dispute resolution in Communist China. *Calif. L. Rev., 55(5)*: 1284–1359.

Ma, Q. (2002) Defining Chinese nongovernmental organizations. *Voluntas: International Journal of Voluntary and Nonprofit Organizations, 13*: 113–130.

Schneider, C. D. (2000) What it means to be sorry: The power of apology in mediation. *Mediation Quarterly, 17*(3): 265–280.

Somers, M. R. (1995) Narrating and naturalizing civil society and citizenship theory: The place of political culture and the public sphere. *Sociological theory*: 229–274.

Perry, E. (2002) Moving the masses: Emotion work in the Chinese Revolution. Mobilization: An International Quarterly, 7(2): 111–128.

Wakeman Jr, F. (1993) The civil society and public sphere debate: Western reflections on Chinese political culture. *Modern China, 19*(2): 108–138.

Yao, Z. (2019) State control and doctors' abuse of clinical autonomy: An empirical analysis of doctors' clinical practice in Chinese public hospitals. *Chinese Journal of Sociology, 5*(1): 29–56.

Yao Zelin. (2015) "Jindai yilai zhongguo yisheng zhiye yu guojia guanxi de yanbian —yizhong zhiye shehuixue de jieshi" ("The Changing Relationship between Chinese Urban Medical Profession and the State since the republican Period: From the perspective of the sociology of professions")*(Sociological Studies)*, (3): 46–68.

Yao Zelin. (2016) "Xingzheng, shichang yu zhiye: chengshi fenji zhenliao de sanzhongzhilimoshi jiqi shijian" ("The evolution of the relationship between the Chinese medical profession and the state in modern times—an explanation from professional sociology") (Social Science), 6: 84–93.

Zhang Jing. (2016) "zhongguo jiceng shehui zhili weihe shixiao?" (Why the grassroots social governance failed) (Zongheng: Quarterly journal of Chinese Thought), *10*.

Appendix A
List of Interview and Interview Script

Appendix A—List of Interview and Interview Script: 2015-2017

a. **Interview List**

	Year 2015	4	
	Year 2016	36	
	Year 2017	32	
Total		72	
By Location			
	City in southern China	5	
	City in east coast of China	5	
	City in northern China	5	
	City in eastern China	57	
Total		72	
Positon			**Avg. Interview Duration (Mins)**
	Bureau of Juridical	5	90
	Government officials	13	30
	Health Care Professionals	29	41.25
	Hospital Manager	3	30
	Medical Disputes Mediation	11	90
	Public Security Department	11	30
Total		72	46.15

b. **Interview Description- For Healthcare Professionals**

- Interview Objective:

J. Wu, *Politicized Medical Dispute Resolution in China*, Understanding China,
https://doi.org/10.1007/978-981-97-6961-2

Interviewee	Objective
Healthcare professionals	•Understand Public Hospital in China •Understand processes in dealing with hospital violence •Understand the government's role in the hospital management

- [Organization] Please describe your organization including number of people, locations and team's role and responsibilities.
- [Organization] What are the key challenges and opportunities for operation in the hospital?
- [Organization] Are there any controls for operations, establishing, communicating, and monitoring policies and procedures? (Interactions with the government)
- [Issue] How much compensation was paid annually for the hospital violence? What's the number of the cases annually in your hospital?
- [Issue] What's the internal process in dealing with hospital violence?
- [Issue] In dealing with hospital violence, what kind of strategies have you applied? E.g. extra internal security, training.
- [Issue] Do you have the experience of dealing with *yinao*? Please elaborate.
- [Issue] Do you think the existing protection from the local government is sufficient to support the internal hospital management on hospital violence?
- [Issue] If no, please identify. If yes, please indicate what kind of protection expected from local government.
- If yes, please indicate what kind of protection received from local government.
- [Reference] Could you recommend your colleague/friend who are suitable for the interview?
- **Interview Description- For Juridical Department – Medical Disputes Mediation Committee**
  - Interview Objective:

Interviewee	Objective
Medical Disputes Mediation Committee	•Understand the organization's objective •Understand processes in dealing with hospital violence •Understand the strategies in the juridical authority in dealing with hospital violence

- [Organization] Please describe your organization including number of people, locations and team's role and responsibilities.
- [Organization] What are the key challenges and opportunities for operation in your organization?

- [Organization] Are there any controls for operations, establishing, communicating, and monitoring policies and procedures? (Interactions with the government)
- [Issue] Why people would choose juridical bureau to solve the hospital violence?
- [Issue] Where does the compensation come from?
- [Issue] Is there any possible that the compensation was credited while the hospital side doesn't do anything wrong?
- [Issue] How's the trust towards your juridical bureau?
- [Issue] How many cases your bureau need to address annually?
- [Issue] What's the trend of the medical disputes?
- [Issue] How's the mediation process (working procedures)?
- [Issue] Have you experienced any hospital violence?
- If yes, could you elaborate?
- If not, could you refer any your colleague who had the experience.
- [Issue] Any typical incident could you share with us?
- [Issue] Do you think the existing protection from the local government is sufficient to support the internal hospital management on hospital violence?
- [Issue] If no, please identify. If yes, please indicate what kind of protection expected from local government.
- If yes, please indicate what kind of protection received from local government.
- [Reference] Could you recommend your colleague/friend who are suitable for the interview?
- **Interview Description- For Public Security Authority**
  - Interview Objective

Interviewee	Objective
Public Security Authority	•Understand the organization's objective •Understand processes in dealing with hospital violence •Understand the strategies in the public security authority in dealing with hospital violence

- [Organization] Please describe your organization including number of people, locations and team's role and responsibilities.
- [Organization] What are the key challenges and opportunities for your organization in addressing the hospital violence?
- [Organization] Are there any controls for operations, establishing, communicating, and monitoring policies and procedures? (Interactions with the government)
- [Issue] How many cases your bureau need to address annually?
- [Issue] How's the mediation process (working procedures)?
- [Issue] Have you experienced any hospital violence?
- If yes, could you describe the scene.
- If not, could you refer any your colleague who had the experience.

- [Issue] Any typical incident could you share with us?
- [Issue] Do you think the existing protection from the local government is sufficient to support the internal hospital management on hospital violence?
- [Issue] If no, please identify. If yes, please indicate what kind of protection expected from local government.
- If yes, please indicate what kind of protection received from local government.
- [Reference] Could you recommend your colleague/friend who are suitable for the interview?

Appendix B

1. Log in the apabi system
   http://www.apabi.com.eproxy2.lib.hku.hk/hku/?pid=usp.search&wd=医闹&cult=TW&db=newspaper&dt=Article&url=usp.search&f_type=&pg=10&dc=2&ps=20 (中华数字书苑)
2. Search the key words: hospital violence (医闹);attack medical workers (伤医).

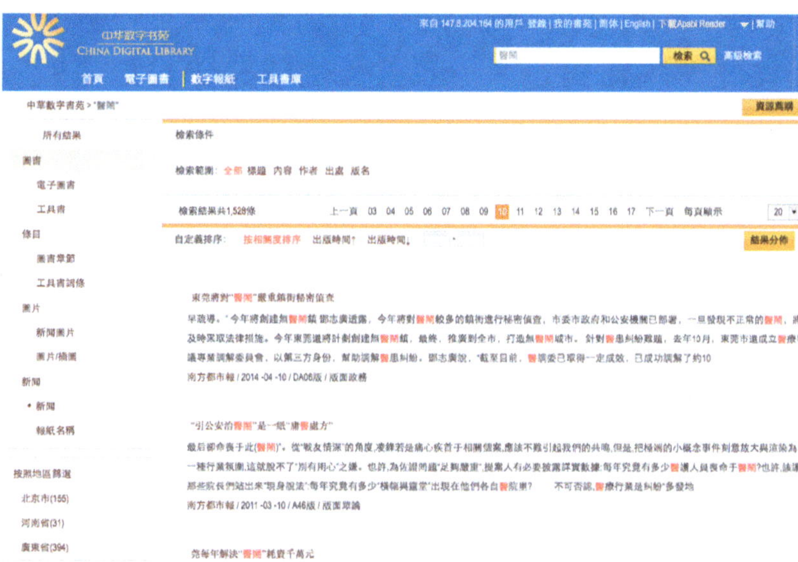

3. There are 1528 news articles in the system. (Duplicate information, 173 remained, among them, only 156 could access with the punishment)
4. Information collection and duplicate check (download)

   - Time of the report (especially pay attention to the words, such as "yesterday")
   - Location of the hospital violence

J. Wu, *Politicized Medical Dispute Resolution in China*, Understanding China,
https://doi.org/10.1007/978-981-97-6961-2

- Hospital information (name, and the level of the hospitals)
- Scale of the hospital violence
- Modes of hospital violence
- Number of casualties
- Reasons
- Punishment: administrative penalty, legal penalty, no penalty

Note: The pictures shown are examples of the data generating process in *chapter 3* from media reports.

Appendix C
Glossary of Chinese Terms

Pinyin	Chinese	English
yinao	医闹	Hospital violence
yiliao jiufen tiaojie weiyuanhui	医疗纠纷调解委员会	Medical dispute mediation committee
tiaojie youxian	调解优先	Mediate first
xinfang	信访	Bureau of letter and visit
nao	闹	Troublemaking
weiwen	维稳	Stability maintenance
hengxiang daobian, zongxiang daodi	横向到边,纵向到底	Horizontal to the edge, vertical in the end
fadong quanshehui yiqilaizuohao weihu shehuiwendinggongzuo	发动全社会一起来做好维护社会稳定工作	Called for a joint effort from all of society to maintain social stability and order
danwei	单位	Work unit system
huatuo	华佗 (人名)	Huatuo
chi jiao yisheng	赤脚医生	Barefoot doctors
baohu san	保护伞	Umbrella of protection
kongbi zheng	空鼻症	Empty nose syndrome
wei quan	维权	Protect rights
wennao	文闹	Non-violent strategies
wunao	武闹	Physical violence
zhongguo renmin zhengzhi xieshang huiyi	中国人民政治协商会议	CPPCC Chinese people's political consultative conference
daye	大爷	Masters
guanxi	关系	Interpersonal relations

(continued)

J. Wu, *Politicized Medical Dispute Resolution in China*, Understanding China,
https://doi.org/10.1007/978-981-97-6961-2

(continued)

Pinyin	Chinese	English
qunti shijian	群体事件	Mass incident
mianzi	面子	Face

MIX
Papier aus verantwortungsvollen Quellen
Paper from responsible sources
FSC® C105338

If you have any concerns about our products,
you can contact us on
ProductSafety@springernature.com

In case Publisher is established outside the EU,
the EU authorized representative is:
Springer Nature Customer Service Center GmbH
Europaplatz 3, 69115 Heidelberg, Germany

Printed by Libri Plureos GmbH
in Hamburg, Germany